My Bubble
Sofia's Story

Becky Meechan

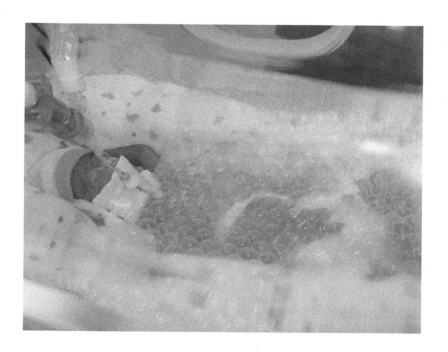

Strategic Book Publishing and Rights Co.

Strategic Book Publishing and Rights Co.
12620 FM 1960, Suite A4-507
Houston, TX 77065
www.sbpra.com

ISBN: 978-1-61897-953-7

Book Design: Suzanne Kelly

This book is dedicated to my precious daughter,
Sofia Angelina Vercesi, born Friday,
February 13, 2009, at 9:32 p.m.,
weighing 1 pound, 8 ounces.

Acknowledgments

There are a number of people who kept me going through the highs and the lows and to this day still remain a tower of strength to me.

Steve, you gave me the most beautiful gift of all, motherhood. Thank you for our beautiful daughter.

Sis, Bren, and Jordy, from across that big old pond, well, what can I say? I love you so much. A sister on a mission is a force to be reckoned with, and thank God I have you as my little sis.

Mom and John, I love you both so much.

Bert, Dange, Vicki, and Les, my closest and dearest friends, you have each provided shoulders for me to sob on, kicked my butt when I doubted my own abilities, and picked me up each time I stumbled and felt weak. Bert, you have endlessly been at my beck and call throughout it all and you have been so instrumental in supporting me write and format the book. You are all my true friends for life!

Rach, my honourary little sister, we love you.

Nanna and Granddad, you are the best and we love you both.

Robert and Sue, thank you for continually picking up the pieces.

Sharon, Bev, and Christine, three incredibly wonderful health visitors, you have been so supportive.

Tracca, Aisha, Deb, and Diane, my wonderful and amazing counselors, if anyone can get you through a breakdown, you are the ladies to do it. You have taught me so much and given me a confidence and belief in myself that I never thought existed.

Dee, you were the one person on the local council that actually made me feel like a human and treated me like one.

Carla, my little fruit bat, you made me laugh so much in SCBU that my sides hurt, and to this day I count you as one of my closest and dearest friends.

Sam and Jackie, you are two wonderful and fantastic nurses.

Jimbo and Kim, you have become close and trusted friends and provided no end of support and help. Jimbo, you have cheered me up a number of times as we put the world to right over a cuppa.

Thank you Mike, the computer wiz who formatted all our images.

Edwina, my little selling machine, thank you for being so active in promoting the book, and thanks to Nina and Sarah for also being so supportive in promoting my book.

To all the friends we made in the hospital, we are the luckiest parents in the world. We also share experiences that have taught us more about the value of life than we could ever learn from a book.

There are many more I would like to thank, and they will all hopefully know how much I regard their friendships and continued support.

To the Little One's that lost their fight for life, you will forever be in our hearts.

Finally, this book would never have been written if it wasn't for the sheer determination to survive against the odds shown by my beautiful daughter. I love you more than words can say, my little Bub.

Introduction

Throughout my adulthood, I'd sit at home and watch commercials for the children's hospitals and wonder to myself, *How on earth do parents cope when they have such sick babies?* The answer is, you just do. Something deep within you kicks in and strength you thought you were never capable of takes over. This strength is tested many times over, but it carries you too—without you even realising it.

When I thought of premature babies I always had this vision of them being just a few weeks early. I never really considered the possibility that babies can be born a number of months early and still survive. When I became pregnant I was not prepared for extreme prematurity; it was more a case of preparation for the slight possibility of having a baby with a disability, given my age of thirty-four.

Being a mommy to an extremely premature baby has been the most harrowing and traumatic experience of my life. Equally so, it has also been the most awakening and rewarding experience.

When my daughter Sofia was born I began a journey of self-discovery, and it taught me the value of the true power of love that exists between a mother and her child.

Unfortunately, to give birth at such an early stage in the pregnancy brings the expectation of doom and gloom, and losing the baby is highly probable. This is a sad fact that you are made painfully aware of. In the early weeks after Sofia's birth, I began to understand that not only do you face a harrowing journey as a family but you also face being ostracised from the ones you least expected it from. As a parent I felt very alone, and I quickly understood that there is very little support for families like ours. It struck me that to receive help you had to go and find it, yet when your child is battling to survive, the last thing you want to do is chase people for support when you should be soothing your little one and encouraging her to keep fighting because Mommy and Daddy so desperately want to take her home. I wanted people to tell me everything would be all right and that one day I would carry my little bundle out of the hospital in a car seat and not a tiny coffin. In those early days, people were unable to give us such reassurance; instead Sofia's fight for life was taken on a day-by-day basis. I was so frightened, too afraid to get my hopes up, as fate had already dealt us so many cruel blows.

Because of this, I made a promise to my angel that one day I would attempt to write her story, in the hope that someday a mommy facing the same journey and feelings of despair would somehow be able to sit down with Sofia's story and hopefully find in it the strength and faith she needs to keep going.

I begin this story with an insight into the slightly traumatic start to my pregnancy, in an attempt to enlighten the reader as to the true battle Sofia faced to survive, because it started even before she was born.

The Journey Begins

For a woman, being pregnant is one of the most amazing and fulfilling roles in life. It is what we do. Or so I thought. My one wish in life was to become a mother, carry a child, give birth, and guide the child through the journey of life.

In September 2008, my wish finally came true. I unexpectedly became pregnant. To say I was ecstatic was an understatement.

I started my pregnancy in a state of disbelief. I wanted to jump, sing, and scream to the world that I was going to be a mommy, but deep down I simply couldn't believe how lucky I was. This feeling of happiness was slightly overshadowed by previous problems that year with my lungs, together with ongoing gynaecological complications, which unfortunately were more likely to cause infertility. I had to face the sad fact that the older I became the further away from becoming a mommy I got. On top of this, there is the little known fact that I have a tendency to be the most jinxed person on this planet! If it's going to happen to anyone, you can bet your bottom dollar it will happen to me! For these reasons alone, I informed my nearest and dearest only of my pregnancy, so as not to tempt fate.

Sadly, within days of my discovery, fate decided to give me a little shake up. I had discharged a large amount of dark blood. My little bubble of joy and happiness burst with an almighty bang. I headed straight to the Accident and Emergency Department of my local general hospital feeling like a broken woman. On arrival at the hospital I somehow managed to explain that I was pregnant and that I thought I had lost my baby—words I never wanted to hear myself saying. I was then whisked off to a room by the nurses to be examined.

Only a minimal physical examination can take place at this stage of the pregnancy because internal examinations can inadvertently cause the loss of a baby if the child has not already passed away. I use the word "baby" at this early stage of my pregnancy because as far as I was concerned the little bundle inside my tummy was already my baby, and I am sure most women would feel the same way.

After what felt like a lifetime in the A and E Department, I was asked to return the following day (due to it being too late in the day) for an ultrasound examination to establish whether or not I was still pregnant. Shaken by the day's events, I went to my mom's house for the night where I spent the longest night of my life (what I later found out would be the first of many) tossing and turning and wanting to go straight back to the hospital and to demand the scan there and then. I was quite confident that I could even do it myself, I was that desperate. Instead, many prayers were said that night and a hell of a lot of begging was done.

The following morning arrived, and I returned to the hospital for the ultrasound scan accompanied by my partner Steve and my mom. While the nurse applied the gel to my tummy and began the scan, I lay on the bed numb and unable to look at the monitor for fear of what she wouldn't find. After what felt like an eternity, I was asked to look at the screen. In front of me I saw the most beautiful sight I'd ever seen in my life. My baby! My tears of sorrow quickly turned into tears of blissful happiness. The baby seemed quite at home in its little den, my little snug bug. The source of the bleeding could not be traced, and so it remained a mystery. We left the hospital and I went home on a high, as a very happy mommy-to-be.

With the blood loss being treated as a threatened miscarriage, I remained off work until after the twelve-week scan. The first trimester is generally considered to be the most vulnerable stage of a pregnancy. With this in mind, it was agreed that I rest for the remainder of this stage.

When we attended the twelve-week scan we were treated to a wave from our cheeky little snug bug, who was happily fidgeting away inside Mommy's tummy.

By twelve weeks I looked very much the pregnant woman! Trying to keep quiet about my pregnancy soon went out the window. I even had "the waddle" due to a previous spinal surgery. I must admit, I loved it; my tummy was growing, as was my baby. I felt "blooming" wonderful.

I returned to work and soon earned the nickname "Dipsy" from the popular children's programme "Teletubbies"—it had something to do with me waddling like a duck and wearing a green sweater. Those gits! So much for keeping a low profile! My work colleagues were as excited as I was at the prospect of a new baby for them to coo over and adore. The affectionate teasing commenced, and my colleagues bustled around looking after the mommy-to-be.

With both my health and pregnancy being a little vulnerable, to say the least, the intention was to take it easy and avoid stress. Unfortunately, my profession was a stressful one; it was that of a forensic scientist. My role was to report DNA findings as an expert witness to the courts in criminal proceedings. Even though I had attended court many times over the years, the anxiety I felt before going onto the stand never left me, and for that reason coupled with the already bumpy start to my pregnancy, I couldn't risk the stress affecting my baby by continuing to appear in court while I was pregnant. Nevertheless, I'd taken quite a bit of time off work that year due to ill health, and one of my pressing court cases had been continually rescheduled pending my return to the office. Out of respect to the court and its consideration of my ill health, I agreed to honour this particular case as my last appearance until after the baby was born. The court was informed of my pregnancy and my recent threatened miscarriage, and a trial date for the case was set.

The day of the court case arrived; it was early on in December 2008. I took along a colleague with the intention that they would be able to witness a criminal court proceeding and observe how we conducted ourselves on the stand. It was good I went with a work buddy, as the weather was so dreadful and the paths were covered in black ice. I'm pretty confident that I looked like a pregnant Bambi on ice as I swung my briefcase around for balance while clutching tightly onto my friend.

We arrived safely at the courthouse, and after sitting around for most of the day, I finally got called to the stand. The case I was testifying in was an armed robbery. As you can imagine, it was of a very serious nature, which in turn meant I would have quite a challenge presenting my evidence on the stand. And I did! Being pregnant and an expert witness does not detract from the severity of a criminal court proceeding. It is nothing personal; you are dealing with people's lives and mistakes cannot be made, therefore the barristers will grill you until they are satisfied you have addressed every point they raised. The grueling questioning finally came to an end, and I was thanked for my evidence and granted permission to leave the courthouse and make my way home. I was absolutely exhausted, both physically and mentally. I was secretly hoping they would give me an easier time. Boy, I was wrong.

Mercifully, the following day I was due to see my consultant, so at least I knew I had the opportunity to recharge my batteries. I also had the comfort of knowing that I had no more court cases to attend for the foreseeable future.

Unfortunately, it transpired that I had made a mistake by agreeing to attend this one last trial. Unbeknownst to me, I had put extra stress on my heart, and because of this I was instructed to remain off work for yet another month due to ill health.

Over the Christmas period I sat dreaming of my next Christmas and looking forward to spending it as a mommy. I also found that as the festive season commenced I craved my favourite foods, including prawns, pâté, and soft cheese—everything a pregnant woman shouldn't be eating! Hormones! Just my luck, only I would crave the foods I could not eat. Whatever happened to cravings of pickled onions and lumps of charcoal? Therefore, while everyone else was tucking into these foods from the gods, I was busy planning a big prawn and pâté feast for next Christmas.

I returned to work at the start of January just as the weather decided it was going to be particularly cold and treacherous underfoot. In mid-January I attended my twenty-week scan and discovered that I was expecting a little girl, who happened to have the legs of a giraffe. Daddy is tall!

At this stage of my pregnancy I had noticed that I was starting to pass a clear, sticky fluid. My instincts were telling me that it was an indication of something nasty. I sought medical advice and was assured it was nothing to worry about and that it was a normal occurrence in pregnancy. Still, it didn't feel right and it continued to concern me.

Toward the end of January the weather had become even more unpleasant, and because I was frightened to death of slipping in the ice and snow, I took a few days leave. In hindsight, I now think it was fate intervening again, but this time it was trying to save my baby; traveling to and from work in normal conditions was a tedious task let alone when the weather was throwing obstacles my way on a daily basis.

January soon moved into February, and I was still passing the clear, sticky fluid.

Then, as if we hadn't had enough to worry about, Friday, February 6th arrived and the nightmare began. I had passed fresh blood. It was a very bad sign. I was informed by the nurses after my threatened miscarriage that fresh blood was a concern that needed to be investigated immediately. Yet again I was rushed off to the hospital. I'd thought the previous threatened miscarriage was a traumatic experience, but this felt a hell of a lot worse. As I sit and write this book two years later, I still struggle to describe the sense of horror and emotional pain I felt at that moment in time.

Because my pregnancy was now further along, the doctors were able to conduct a slightly uncomfortable but necessary internal examination. My cervix was intact and they were unable to source the cause of the bleeding, so yet again I was sent home and told to rest. It wasn't as if I'd been exerting myself while the weather was bad anyway; I'd been fixed in front of the TV enjoying daytime television and the best comedy in the world: "Only Fools and Horses" with the occasional Jeremy Kyle thrown in. Who doesn't enjoy that?

Saturday passed with a smaller amount of blood being lost, but it was still fresh and I continued to feel that something was very wrong. Part of me was hoping it was a good sign that the blood loss had begun to diminish. Wishful thinking!

Sunday arrived and my worst fears were confirmed. Steve was busy collecting furniture from my mom and stepfather, John, while I busied myself with the Sunday dinner. I had just taken the chicken out of the oven (it's funny the things you remember) and I needed to use the toilet. So off I went, only to discover that I had passed a very large amount of fresh blood and what also appeared to be the mucus plug, which I knew to be normally discharged while giving birth. I called my mom and she rushed over and took me straight back to the hospital.

Somehow I knew that this time it was going to be very, very bad.

On arrival at the hospital, I went straight into a room in the maternity unit and prepared for another internal examination. I lay on the bed absolutely terrified as my mom tried to console me. Finally, a doctor and nurse came into my room and explained that they were going to examine my cervix again.

As they began my examination, I witnessed the lightning-quick look they exchanged, and as they both rose from the end of my hospital bed I knew it was bad news. I felt my world fall apart. With dire expressions on their faces, they broke the news that would change my life forever.

At just twenty-four weeks into my pregnancy my amniotic sac had prolapsed though my cervix. I had an incompetent cervix, meaning my baby decided she was going to make an exceptionally early appearance, and because of this it was highly likely that she would pass away. All I ever dreamed of in life was becoming a mommy, and now it felt like my baby was being taken from me in the cruelest way possible.

Words cannot describe the devastation I felt at that moment. I felt pain and emotion swell from deep inside me as I sobbed and pleaded for my baby to live. My mom tried to comfort me and then called Steve to get him to come straight to the hospital. But how can you comfort a woman who has just been told that her baby is coming too early and has very little chance of survival?

I was also informed that I had only just reached the "viable" stage of my pregnancy, which is hospital talk for recognising a baby as a human with the right to life. Therefore, they had to do what they could to save the baby's life when born at this stage of the pregnancy. In all honesty, I believe that even if the baby came before the twenty-four week stage the hospital would still have tried their hardest to save her life. I lay in the bed numb, listening as they explained to us what was going to happen. My bed was tilted, in attempt to encourage gravity to pull the prolapsed amniotic sac back into my womb. If successful, this would allow them to attempt to put a stitch into my cervix. This procedure would be performed with the intention of trying to prolong the pregnancy to a more viable stage in which the baby could be born with a greater chance of survival. It was a risky procedure in this situation, but if successful that little stitch could be the difference between life and death for my daughter.

I was then informed that the hospital I was at was not a specialist hospital, which meant that they had the facilities to deliver the little one but not to keep her alive; this would necessitate a specialist neonatal unit.

It was arranged for a paediatric consultant to visit me and discuss the life expectancy of my baby and explain to me in more detail the battle she would face if she were to survive.

In all honesty, a lot of what was happening around me was a complete blur; I was in a daze and absolutely devastated. I just wanted my baby to live, and yet everyone was telling me that she was going to have one hell of a fight for survival on her tiny little hands. As they continued to talk to me I felt I was being prepared for the death of my daughter.

Steve soon arrived at the hospital, and when the extent of the situation was explained to him he too looked like his world had just fallen apart. He phoned his parents and told them to come straight to the hospital.

I was informed by the doctor that I was to have two steroid injections straight into the muscles of my thighs. The steroid acts like a life-support fluid. It is injected into the mommy's body but passes through to the baby's body in an attempt to give her tiny underdeveloped lungs a chance at life when she is born. The injection has to be given in two doses twelve hours apart. There is no guarantee the steroid will work, but it is the best chance the baby has when faced with a life-threatening situation such as extreme prematurity.

We had a visit from the paediatric consultant, who reiterated the news that little one was in a life-threatening position and that the odds were stacked against her survival but they would endeavor to try and save her life. I wanted to hear things like, "No problem, we see this all the time and the babies are all fit and well and at home before you know it," yet those words never came. Instead, there were looks of pity and helplessness, nothing that gave us hope.

A bed was arranged for Steve so he could spend the night at my side; it was understood that the baby could arrive at any moment, especially as it was looking more and more unlikely that the prolapsed sac would return to a safe position.

I was given the first steroid. Never before had I hoped and prayed so much to make it through the next twelve hours to get a second injection. I knew this steroid could be the difference between life and death for our baby, and as each second of the clock passed excruciatingly slow I knew that no matter what, we had to make it to the second steroid if the little one was going to have any chance of survival.

Until that night, I never really appreciated just how slow time is. I remember drifting in and out of sleep and looking at the clock only to find it had hardly moved. At one point during the night as I lay on my side facing away from Steve, I heard this startled noise arise from him. Apparently he had turned over in his bed and was faced with the sight of my naked bottom poking out of the sheets. It still makes me giggle to this day.

Finally, night turned into day and I was given the second steroid injection. The relief I felt was overwhelming. I honestly believed that my baby had been given a little bit more hope. I was also ecstatic that she had survived yet another life-threatening night.

As my obstetrics consultant was based at the hospital, I asked that he be informed about the situation the minute he arrived at work. He had been treating me for my gynaecological problems since my university days and we had become close over the years. I knew that he too would be devastated at the news, but I also knew that he would do whatever he could to save my daughter. Mid-morning, in between his theater list, he arrived at my bedside. I trusted this man with both our lives, and he didn't let us down.

A meeting was held and specialist hospitals all over the country were contacted to ascertain their bed availability. We had one slight problem: Being transported was going to be a very dangerous procedure for both our lives. Because the amniotic sac had prolapsed, there was the distinct possibility that the slightest bump could trigger labour, and being transported in an ambulance in a situation that required highly trained specialists from both the surgical and paediatric areas was going to take some serious planning. It would also mean racing against time. It felt like an impossible situation; it would be safer for both of us to be together and moved as one, but moving us was the dangerous part. Even the air ambulance was ruled out of the equation because it was considered too dangerous.

While the meeting was underway, my mom, John, and Steve's parents arrived back at the hospital, all thankful that we had made it through the first night.

Finally, a decision was made by the medical team and preparations for our transfer were put into place. I was to be moved to a nearby specialist hospital, which fortunately had a bed for us. This sounds like a simple enough transfer procedure, but unfortunately the complexity of the situation required that a specialist neonatal nurse, midwife, and anaesthetist had to be part of the transfer from hospital to hospital to cover all eventualities. This then resulted in a delay with the transfer, because it was a "timed transfer." A timed transfer is when a specific time is set so all the specialists who are involved can clear their schedules and meet at the designated time to ensure that the transfer can proceed safely and smoothly. My consultant had stated categorically that unless all of the professionals were available at the given time then I could not be moved. The journey was planned. I was to be in the first ambulance with the specialist neonatal nurse, a paramedic, and the driver. A paramedic vehicle would carry the emergency team and a neonatal ventilator (life support machine) and a further ambulance with an emergency team, and a second neonatal ventilator would also be set up and ready to meet us en route to the receiving hospital in case I went into labour and they had to pull over and perform emergency surgery. To finish off this true cannonball run-style manoeuvre, the remainder of the convoy was composed of Steve in one car, my mom and John in a second car, and Steve's parents in the third car.

I never knew there were so many different routes to take in one direction.

Apparently when we left the hospital, Steve was glued to the back of my ambulance; he was not letting us out of his sight! While everyone else spread out the minute they left the hospital grounds. Each driver convinced they knew the quickest route. How we all arrived at our destination at more or less the same time still puzzles me to this day.

On arrival at our new hospital, I was taken straight to a room and resumed my 'bat' like position, feet above my head level. While the others discussed their journey adventures, the nursing staff scanned my tummy for signs that the little one was still okay.

Finally I was settled and my new medical team approached me.

A female consultant approached the small group gathered around my bedside and made what is to be considered not the most sensitive of comments: "You are all looking miserable!" It was also not the wisest of comments to make in front of a man whose partner and a child were in a life-threatening situation. Steve replied, "No, wrong word. Not 'miserable,' 'worried.'" Considering the severity of the situation, it was to be expected!

It is hard to put your trust in someone who makes such insensitive remarks at a time when a family is facing its worst fears.

Again, we were visited by various people, all reiterating the same information we had already been provided with at the previous hospital. However, this time in my room I had a baby ventilator (life support machine). It was a stark reminder of what was to come.

At some point I was moved into the delivery suite. Because the amniotic sac was still prolapsed I was to remain in my bat-like position, hooked up to drips and continually subjected to blood tests. It soon became evident that my body was not working as it should have been. I was showing signs of some form of infection, but it could not be sourced and my blood pressure and heart rate were all to pot too. Mentally I was in turmoil and absolutely petrified for my daughter's life. In myself, I didn't feel ill. However, I did have a very strange sense of peacefulness hanging over me. I genuinely felt that it didn't matter what happened to me as long as my little one was safe; Daddy would always worship her and love her. We asked that they continually listen for her heartbeat. We needed to hear her; it was important for us to hear our girl. Steve even recorded the sound of the baby's heart beating away on his mobile phone. Throughout all of this, each time the scan was performed, we found ourselves holding our breaths while they struggled to trace the little one's whereabouts in my body in order to detect her heartbeat. Then as soon as we heard that little *whoosh whoosh* of the baby's heart, I couldn't help but burst into tears. My little fighter! We later discovered that it was so difficult to pick up her heartbeat because she was trapped inside the birth canal, and being so tiny it was incredibly difficult to track her down. They would have had more luck searching for the Scarlet Pimpernel!

As the journey between hospitals had been successful and my condition seemed stable, I was moved into a room to rest and await the impending birth of my little one. Yet again, wherever my bed was put, so was the baby's life support machine.

Over the next couple of days visitors came and went. I remained bed-bound and elevated. Steve fed me because my hands had IV drips in them, which made it painful and difficult to move them. Even the menial task of me sitting up in bed could be enough to trigger labour. I just lay in my room and watched as life went on around me.

Steve and I continually asked for the scan to be carried out so we could hear our little one; it was all we had to hold on to, the sound of her little heartbeat. Each time the scan was performed, it took a while to locate our tiny daughter's heartbeat, and each time we held our breaths until we heard the little beating heart of our girl! You see, our little one's heartbeat told us so much. It was strong! This meant she was showing signs of strength too, which is what she desperately needed to stay alive.

Wednesday passed, and the situation had not improved. My blood was still continually being tested and we continued listening for her heartbeat. Emotionally, I was up and down. One minute I was sobbing, the next I was trying to pull myself together because I was so frightened of upsetting the baby and distressing her. I had to try so hard to be positive and hold it together.

Steve and I formed a bond with our nurses, who were incredibly supportive. We would share jokes and chat, anything to not face the horrors of what was happening. Still I remained unhappy with the consultant; she had lost my trust and respect with her initial comment, and for that I simply could not take to her. I dreaded her visits and the anticipation of what she would say next.

Thursday arrived. It was around midday and I had sent Steve home for a rest, feeling that because nothing had happened since Sunday we were safe. Steve was exhausted and I was relying on him to be physically and emotionally strong for when the baby came. While lying in bed as usual, I suddenly had the very strange feeling of a falling sensation come from within my tummy, even with my legs raised above my head. Due to my tummy being swollen I had lost sight of my feet since being bed-bound and I was unable to work out what was happening. I felt no pain but I knew something was amiss. I buzzed for the nurses. They came into my room and I explained to them what had just happened as they lifted the sheet from my body. Again, people really do need to work on their facial expressions when dealing with a shocking sight. Like before, I knew something bad had happened just by observing their reactions. It was very bad; I lay in a pool of blood.

I had to be moved immediately to the birthing suite. It looked like my little one was coming. I called Steve in tears and told him to come straight back to the hospital and that I was losing large amounts of blood. I was actually haemorrhaging.

By the time the equipment was set up around me, Steve was back at my bedside. The consultant came into the room and explained to us that she appeared to be making her way. With the haemorrhaging as bad as it was, both Steve and I were terrified that our baby was in danger. After voicing our fears we were informed by the consultant that my baby would die inside my body if she didn't come out soon because they considered my life to be more important. Again, this was not an appropriate comment to make to two extremely distressed parents-to-be. I begged for them to scan me again; we wanted to hear her little heartbeat. I asked for them to do a Caesarean section in order for my daughter to have a chance. I was informed that this was not possible at this stage of the pregnancy because it was too dangerous a procedure for me to undergo. I sobbed and sobbed. How could she be so clinical? I really didn't care about any damage to my body; I just wanted my daughter to have a chance. How could they let my baby die inside? I lay there while Steve tried to comfort me, and as hard as I tried not to, I couldn't help but sob. Meanwhile, the blood continued to pool on my bed.

Steve spoke with the nurses and said he would take over collecting the pooling blood and huge blood clots as they passed out of my body. He told them that he would continue to clean my body because he felt he needed to be involved in looking after us. A stainless steel trolley was set up at the side of my bed. Steve was to place all the blood-saturated clinical towels onto this trolley. They were trying to monitor the extent of the blood loss from my body. No sooner had he cleared away the blood-stained towels and cleaned me than I was saturated again. All night long he tended to me, not once complaining or letting me know the extent of the horrors he was seeing. He would just lean over, kiss me, and tell me to try and sleep. Every couple of hours the nurses would pop in and scan my tummy so we could hear a certain little person's heartbeat.

By Friday morning the bleeding had started to calm down and I was moved into yet another room to rest and await the arrival of my little one. Again my daughter's trusty life support machine followed me.

At around lunchtime, I told Steve to go home again for a rest; he was looking absolutely washed out. I have since learned not to send him home, as it clearly means everything will go pear-shaped the minute he leaves my side.

Again, Steve had already left hospital, and yet again I experienced another falling sensation from inside my tummy. Thinking it was another huge blood clot, I told my mom, who had arrived to take over from Steve, and she called for the nurses. But this time when they examined me even my mom had that "Oh my God" look on her face. The amniotic sac that my little one was held in had dropped through my body and was hanging out of me looking like a wobbly Easter egg. It was a sac of murky-coloured fluid with the umbilical cord bobbing around inside it. I am glad I never saw this sight because the looks on everybody's faces told me just how horrific it was.

Steve didn't even make it home before he received a phone call urgently telling him to come back.

This time there was no mistaking it: My little one was coming. The gas and air were hooked up and I was put into the birthing position. I was incredibly weak and tired. I hadn't even started attending antenatal classes yet; I was only just getting to that stage of my pregnancy. I had absolutely no idea how on earth I was supposed to do things. I was being told to push, and push I did. Well, I thought I was pushing. But surprisingly enough I had no feeling whatsoever down below. I had not even had an epidural. I think this lack of feeling was simply because my daughter was so tiny that my body didn't even really register that she was trying to escape. All I remember at the time is a crippling pain shooting through the area of my spine, which

I'd previously had surgery on. Everybody was saying words of encouragement and telling me to push, and I was crying because I was pushing so hard and couldn't even feel anything. Apparently, the amniotic sac had prolapsed further out of my body, but each time I rested due to exhaustion it began to retract again. The gas and air did absolutely nothing. I'm sure I told them that I thought the machine was faulty; I simply didn't feel that it had any effect whatsoever on me. Steve decided to have a go on the gas and air himself and he was happy it was working well enough; he stayed on it long enough to be convinced.

Time passed and I continued to push and push, but to no avail. The medical team was beginning to show signs of concern. They informed us that they needed to carry out an ultrasound scan to see why the baby was not coming out. In theory she should have literally popped out. The portable scanner was wheeled into my room and we were all eager to find out what the baby was up to. At this point I discovered that my daughter was already demonstrating that she had inherited some of my traits. Not wanting to make things easy for herself, my little baby had decided she wanted to have an adventure and be different by coming out feet first. Again, this was an incredibly dangerous situation for both of us to be put in. A new consultant had come on duty for the weekend and he was now to be overseeing us. He turned to us and explained that our little one still had a strong heartbeat, but unfortunately she was trapped in a breach position and in turn this meant that if we were to continue with a natural birth, she would die because my cervix was only dilated by 5 centimeters. Because the labour was progressing in a very dangerous way, a senior consultant had also been called in to assist. Given the comments made previously by the original female consultant, Steve and I became very distressed at this news. I again begged for them to try and save my girl and pleaded for them to perform a Caesarean section. To which they both replied, "Of course we will." We didn't expect that. I was so happy they didn't patronise us but instead promised they would do their utmost to save our girl.

Firstly we had to discuss the severity of the surgery given the complications we had already faced. I didn't care what they did to me; I just wanted my baby to have a chance. I was not giving up on her now.

It was decided that I would be given an epidural, and then if necessary I could be fully anesthetised. We were informed that only Steve would be allowed into the operating theatre with me. Finally my bed was wheeled into the operating theatre and Steve was taken away to be gowned up.

It wasn't the looks the looks on people's faces that startled me this time, it was the cry of "Oh my God" from an operating theatre nurse as I was wheeled in lying on my side with a fluid-filled bulge hanging from my body. People really need to think before they speak! It was at that moment I suddenly realised how horrific our situation was. The sight of my body had shocked a professional nurse so much that she cried out in alarm.

The operating theatre team quickly gathered around me and started to utter words of reassurance and comfort, and as I turned my head and looked over to the doorway, in walked six-foot-odd "Fifi the Flower Fairy." It was Steve. I laughed. He had on a yellow surgical hat all puffed up around his head and a green operating gown. It was such a comical sight.

The anaesthetist approached me and explained that I would have to curl up as much as possible on my side as he adminis-tered the anaesthetic. Boy, did it hurt. I was also very frightened that the sac would burst as I lay scrunched up. He skillfully inserted the needle into my spine and then I was repositioned onto my back. A drape was put up over my tummy so that we had no sight of the horrors they were about to uncover. After a few minutes the anaesthetist carried out a series of tests all over my body to establish if I was numb. It worked; he was absolutely brilliant. He positioned himself at the top of my head, ready to put me under full anaesthetic at the drop of a hat. Steve was seated to my right. In the far corner of the room the paediatric consultants waited and began preparing the life support machine and equipment for our little one. My ventilator was on my left, should I need it. Finally, on either side of my abdomen stood a surgeon and the remainder of their team.

The procedure began. Steve held my hand tightly; he kept giving me little kisses and whispering to me, telling me we were all going to make it through this. While the surgeons began to work on me, Steve and I tried to decide on our little one's name. Anything to try and soften the gravity of the situation we were in. We had narrowed the baby's name down to Fiorella or Sofia. As I lay there with my body being pulled to and fro we finally decided on Fiorella, "little flower." We had already chosen the baby's middle name and it was to be Angelina without a shadow of doubt because the name means "little angel." We wanted every bit of spiritual help we could get.

At one point I remember us all laughing because one of the consultants admitted that he hadn't even planned for Valentine's Day, which was the following day, and he was trying to work out where to get flowers at that time of night. We had a fantastic team working on us and everybody in that operating theatre tried their hardest to distract me from becoming overwhelmed, and to be honest it worked.

I knew that behind that screen a surgeon's nightmare was unfolding. My body was being lifted and pulled, and I could see the concern in Steve's face each time I was visibly lifted from the bed. Each time he saw the panic rising in my eyes he tried incessantly to stop it and keep me calm. I was later told of the difficulties the team had faced.

Finally, Steve suddenly looked up at me and asked, "Did you just hear that?" Dazed, I asked him what he meant and he told me that he had just heard a tiny little squeak. Moments later everything went a bit crazy. The baby had been removed from my body and she was now lying in the life support machine out of sight while they fought to save her life. The repair work on my body began while my little one was cleaned and wrapped in bubble wrap and hooked up to the baby life support machine. Before the work was finished on me, we were informed that our baby was ready to be moved into the intensive care unit. Slowly the machine that had been stalking me for days was wheeled past us, and the tiniest little bundle I had ever seen in my life was lying in the centre of it. The doctor pulled back the cover and revealed the side of my daughter's teeny little head; it was the size of a hen egg. I remember crying out that she looked just like daddy; even at this stage she was his little double. We then both sobbed as they took my baby from me; I knew it had only just begun and that I may never hold her alive. How can someone so tiny and fragile possibly survive?

While the surgeons finished operating on me, Steve left the operating theatre. He was told that he would be able to go and visit our little one in the Bliss intensive care unit as soon as she was settled and me in the adult intensive care unit when I was stabilised.

Our beautiful baby daughter was born at 9:32 p.m. on Friday, February 13, 2009 (yes, Friday the 13th!), weighing only 1 pound, 8 ounces. My tiny "Polly Pocket."

Eventually, I was wheeled out of the operating theatre and moved into intensive care. I had lost a large amount of blood and my body was exhausted, as was my mind. While I was stabilised, Steve, my mom, and John all went to see our beautiful little daughter.

When they at last walked into my room, their eyes were full of tears. Steve walked up to my bed and kissed me. He then said, "She's a Sofia; she's dark and she's beautiful." So Sofia (meaning "wisdom") it was. My beautiful baby daughter, Sofia Angelina Vercesi. She won't thank us for that one when she has to spell it. They went on to tell me how incredibly tiny she was and that her teeny little hands were trying to grab the bubble wrap that she lay in. Daddy was so amazed and so proud of her. I couldn't stop crying. I couldn't see my baby, I couldn't smell her, I couldn't hold her, and I couldn't kiss her. My poor, tiny baby was battling for her life and her mommy couldn't even be with her!

We were told that the next twenty-four hours were critical for Sofia. If she made it through them, then we would look at the next forty-eight hours and so on. This was not quite what I had expected to be faced with when I discovered I was pregnant and eagerly awaiting the birth of my child.

We were visited by the surgeons, who explained that my body had taken a tremendous battering throughout the surgery, as did Sofia's. She was heavily bruised when they pulled her from my tummy. She was so badly trapped inside me that my womb had to be lifted and split in half in an attempt to get to her. On top of that, the placenta was also blocking access to her, which made the procedure even more complicated. Throughout the surgery I had also lost a tremendous amount of blood, which had pooled inside my abdomen. I had a tube running from my tummy into a drainage bag to try and remove the remainder of the blood that had filled my body. Unbelievably, though, the surgeons informed us that they had saved my womb, and although I could never give birth to another child, it was likely that I could have another baby with surgical intervention at both the start and end of the pregnancy. They were fantastic surgeons, and gentlemen too.

Finally, at some point during the early hours, everyone left me to rest and I dropped off into a morphine-induced, exhausted sleep.

Somewhere in the hospital my baby's fight for survival had only just began.

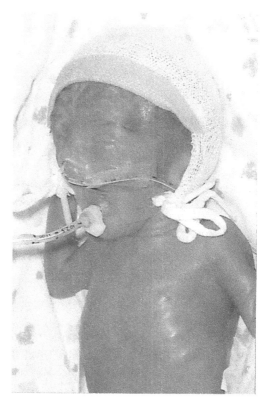

This is the very first picture taken of Sofia and it was taken by the staff in the Bliss intensive care unit. This enabled Mommy to see her beautiful baby. Sofia's skin has a shiny, waxy appearance to it.

19

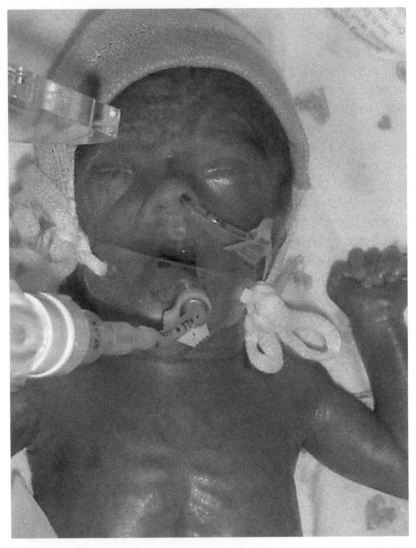

This picture was taken by a very proud daddy. Sofia's eyes are still sealed shut and the life support tube is going through her mouth and into her lungs. The nasal gastric tube is fed through Sofia's nose.

This was the beginning of an emotional journey full of tears, anger, frustration, pain, laughter, and the most wonderful bond of love.

Sofia's Fight for Life

The day after Sofia was born I was allowed to visit her. I was still heavily under the influence of morphine and still in a state of shock as to what had happened.

I remember being wheeled down a corridor not wanting to make eye contact with people. I felt like a failure. My baby was fighting for her life because my body couldn't carry her.

I was taken down a long corridor and we came to a halt outside a room named "Bliss" about halfway down. Unfortunately, as we were about to enter the room in which Sofia was now living, I looked down and saw a trail of blood. It was from me. My hand was bleeding quite badly from the wound left by my IV drip. So instead of going in to see Sofia we had to turn back and get my hand redressed. Not a good start.

Finally, we returned to the corridor outside Sofia's new home. I was wheeled into a room full of incubators and bleeps and all sorts of equipment and noises, and I had absolutely no idea where my baby was. Slowly my wheelchair was pushed forward toward this little plastic baby greenhouse and there inside laid my incredibly tiny daughter. She would have fit inside my hand. I had never seen a baby so small and fragile before in my life. I burst into tears and told them to take me away. I couldn't do it! I couldn't look at my daughter. I had never seen a baby born so premature. I couldn't get my head around the fact that I should never have seen my daughter at this stage of my pregnancy outside my body and just how different she looked from what I had expected when I first became pregnant. All I could think was that I had done this to her. I couldn't hold her in my body and protect her and now she was lying there with tubes sticking out from her tiny, battered and bruised body, and it was all my fault.

I looked at her and wondered how she could possibly survive. She looked so frail; even her skin looked as if it would tear at the slightest touch. I broke down and sobbed. I didn't see how there could be a light at the end of the tunnel. I genuinely believed there was no way my daughter would make it. What chance did a baby born this early have? I was too afraid to love her. I knew I would never be able to deal with the loss of her if she didn't make it. I felt that while she was in my body I was keeping her safe and now I had to rely on others and trust them to do my job.

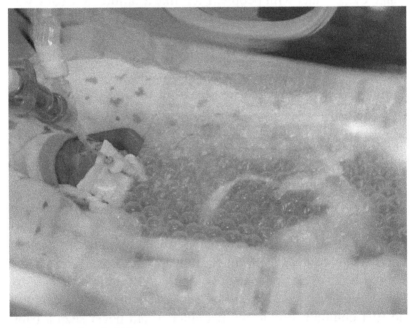

Sofia encased up bubble wrap

Again, all around me people looked at me with knowing eyes. They knew Sofia would need a miracle to survive; she was just too early, and they knew they were a looking at a woman who may never take her child home and may never hear her daughter's laughter as she grows up.

The First Week

Initially I was moved into an open ward full of new moms and their babies, but after my mother pointed out the insensitivity of this move to the staff I was transferred into a private room.

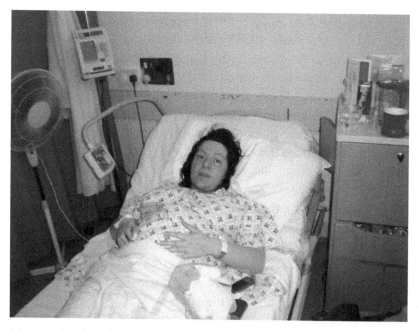

Mommy, the day after Sofia's birth after coming out of the adult intensive care unit

It took a few days for the drugs to work their way out of my body and for me to be able to sit with Sofia for any length of time. As the hours passed I couldn't help but fall deeply in love with my daughter. I became determined to make sure she knew who her mommy was and how much she loved her. I knew that apart from my being able to produce milk for her, all I could do now was talk to her, touch her, and show my love for her because I was not giving up on my girl, not now, not after everything we had gone through together. Sofia was going to know without a shadow of a doubt just how much Mommy loved her and how determined Mommy was to take her home no matter what.

Admittedly, I was also an absolute wimp at this stage. I was terrified of touching Sofia in case I hurt her or accidentally knocked one of the multiple tubes sticking out from her tiny body.

Within days of Sofia's birth I had to learn to express my milk. Again, my body wasn't ready for this and it was a daunting situation to be faced with; I knew how crucial a mother's milk was to a newborn, let alone one that was critically ill and fighting for her life. Apparently it is also very common for mommies of twenty-four-week-old babies to "dry up" and not be able to maintain their milk supply. Having this knowledge made me even more anxious. I personally felt that replacing my baby with a mechanical pump was as far away from feeling the touch and warmth of my own child nursing as I could get. But I was a mommy on a mission. After some perseverance with my little "C3P0" milking machine I produced a tiny drop of milk, just 3 milliliters (less than a teaspoon). I was so happy but also so disappointed because I had naively expected to produce at least a pint. It turned out that my tiny little drop would actually provide Sofia with a few feedings.

We were told that having your baby near you when expressing helps with milk production. Unfortunately my baby was in a life support incubator and I had to express my milk in an old cupboard down the corridor from the Bliss room. Steve and I nicknamed it the "milking cupboard." It was so tiny that only one mommy could use it at any given time. You couldn't even swing a rat in it let alone a cat. Each day I would await my turn then disappear off to the cupboard and express my milk. I was so desperate to keep it flowing because in my eyes it was my only valuable contribution as a mommy to keeping my daughter alive.

In order for Sofia to have a feeding, which was literally a tiny drop of my milk, a test had to be carried out on her stomach contents. It was an acidity (pH) test. Because Sofia was born too early, her organs were not fully developed; her eyes hadn't even opened yet. A feeding tube (nasal gastric tube) was fed through one of her minute nostrils and into her stomach so that any fluids could be administered directly without her needing to swallow. Sofia's body had yet to learn the art of pushing food from one end to the other (known as peristalsis). However, as with many procedures used on extremely premature babies, with this method of feeding comes the very dangerous threat of the tube slipping out of the stomach and into the lungs. This can happen, believe me. Milk in the lungs could result in death (the lungs would be filled with fluid), especially as Sofia's lungs were not even fully formed yet. In order for us to be certain that the tube was safely housed we had to carry out the pH test each time anything was administered down her feeding tube, whether it be medication or milk. If the reaction indicated acidity then that was the green light that everything was safe and we were able to continue, as this verified that the tube was correctly positioned inside our little one's stomach. If the reaction came back as neutral then further testing would need to be carried out because a neutral reaction could also be caused by previous milk still being undigested. We needed to ensure the tube hadn't slipped out of the baby's stomach and into her lungs, which would also give a neutral result. Whenever we were uncertain we called for assistance from one of the nurses. We were just not taking the risk.

After being taught how to feed Sofia by the nurses, I made Steve do the first feeding because I was just so frightened that I would harm her. On a good day I am clumsy so in times of anxiety I am lethal, and she was so unbelievably fragile.

It took me several weeks before I felt comfortable carrying out this pH test. I was convinced that I was going to suck Sofia's tummy out with the syringe because quite often when you perform this test there is quite a lot of resistance. It felt like we were subjecting our baby to cruelty.

Each day we sat at Sofia's bed side chatting to her and watching her, too frightened to do anything. We learned to give her baby bed baths (known as All Care), which involved using sterile water to wipe over her face and body. We would apply a little "lip gloss" with a sterile cotton wool bud, which was simply some Vaseline on her lips, as they would become very dry. We also did little nappy changes too. Again, I am happy to admit that I am naïve. Sofia's external genitalia and bottom cheeks had not yet developed. I just assumed that meant she was unable to wee and poo. But I was wrong. Sofia's first little poo made us so proud because we just didn't expect it. She was extremely fussy about being in a mess too. Because Sofia was too tiny, at first she lay on top of her miniscule nappy so we were able see immediately if she had done a little poo. If so, we had to clean her promptly because she would try and lift her body from the nappy. She seemed to get very upset. It was the most fascinating sight to witness when she raised her tiny fragile body; at the same time, it also terrified us. We were so convinced that she would harm herself with the tubes. Where on earth does that strength come from?

Each day we had our little family duties in order for us to bond and show our girl that her parents were there at her bedside. We were desperate for her to know just how much we loved her.

Throughout the first week Sofia had to undergo ultraviolet treatment (phototherapy). Her liver was underdeveloped, which in turn meant it was not able to perform its tasks as efficiently as a full-term baby. As a consequence of this, she developed jaundice. This is a condition in which the skin appears to have a yellowish tinge to it, and it occurs because of an increase in a substance called bilirubin. Bilirubin is chemical produced by the body to break down old red blood cells. Phototherapy treatment has been found to reduce the levels of bilirubin in the body. Sofia also had only a small amount of blood in her body, which caused her to be severely anaemic too. To try and build up her blood capacity and strength, she underwent a number of blood transfusions. Sofia's body was also unable to make its own blood. Sofia was battling septicaemia (a bacterial infection that enters the bloodstream and can result in death) so she began receiving antibiotics to try and combat it. Sofia also had bleeding on the brain; again, this is common when babies are born so premature. Sofia needed to have a number of scans and X-rays on various parts of her body to try and establish exactly how well she was coping outside Mommy's tummy. Her lungs were clearly underdeveloped and struggling, especially as they were continually filled with fluid.

Caffeine was used to help with Sofia's breathing difficulties; it has been found to help regulate breathing in babies as premature as Sofia. She also had a duct in her heart that had not yet closed. While Sofia battled hard for life, her underdeveloped organs struggled to work. Any lines going into her hands/arms and feet/legs were supported by tiny little splints, which made it even harder to touch Sofia and for her to move comfortably; she looked like she was covered in tiny surfboards. On top of all this, Sofia's weight had dropped too. After a few days on life support Sofia was then put onto biphasic CPAP (Continuous Positive Airway Pressure) because she was coping on her own a little bit. This system is the next step down from life support, and instead of the machine doing all the work the baby has a little go too, and when she becomes weak or too tired it helps take away the burden of trying to breathe on her own.

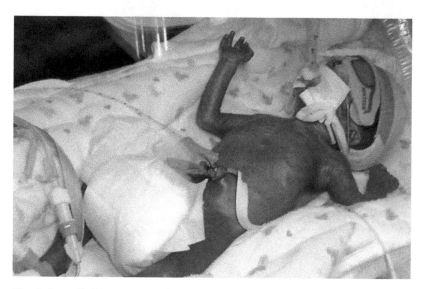

Newly born Sofia receiving phototherapy while lying on top of her nappy. The umbilicus is the most effective way of administering medication into a baby as tiny as Sofia because her veins were incredibly minuscule and fragile.

Steve and I gradually began to learn the functions of all the machines and their different alarm sounds and what they each meant, and also the drugs being used to keep Sofia alive. Steve had borrowed the mother of all drug books from a friend who worked in the medical field and each time a new drug was introduced he made a note of it and researched it when he got home. He wanted to know exactly what was being pumped into his baby's little body and why.

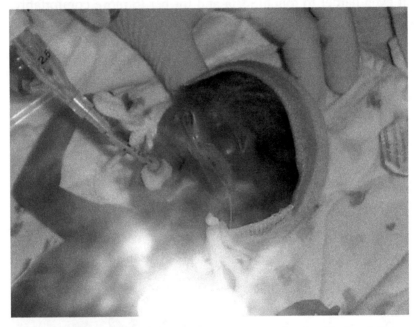

You can see how small Sofia was in comparison to the size of a hand. Her little head was the size of a hen egg.

Sofia's Daily Battle

From this point onward I kept a daily record of Sofia's battles while in hospital. Some days are more detailed than others, and some days were harder to face than others. I didn't always remember to put everything down; Sofia underwent many procedures, but I tried to capture what I could. It's only now as I think back that I remember how this became our norm. Each day our baby would undergo painful tests and treatments needed to keep her alive, and each day we would watch as our daughter fought to live.

One Week Old

February 20—Seven days old

Sofia has opened her right eye, and what a beautiful little eye it is.

Sofia's little personality is beginning to show and she continues to grasp at anything she can get her tiny hands on, including all the wires and tubes attached to her. Little monkey!

I tube-fed Sofia for the first time today and changed her little nappy. It was very scary for me, and I couldn't stop shaking. I got a kick for that.

February 21—Eight days old

Today Daddy fed Sofia and carried out her baby bed bath for the first time. Daddy also changed a very dirty nappy. He was brilliant and Sofia seemed to love it, as she lay there quite relaxed and content.

February 22—Nine days old (26th week of gestation)

Sofia is now showing signs of her left eye opening, and now she is trying to follow Daddy and I as we move around outside her little home.

One thing that we have discovered about Sofia is that our little girl really doesn't like a dirty nappy and becomes very distressed when she has one. Sofia digs her little feet into her bedding and then arches her body up like a little crab.

Sofia does not like being handled because she is hypersensitive to touch and she's not afraid to let the doctors and nurses know, usually by having a teeny temper tantrum whereby she will kick out those little legs and thrash around those little noodle arms. Uncle Bren has nicknamed Sofia his "little noodle" after seeing how tiny her little arms are.

Poppet can now wrap her tiny fingers around the tips of our little fingers and every now and again she gives us a tiny squeeze.

Sofia also makes the cutest baby noises in the world; if we stand right next to her incubator and open one of the doors we can just about hear her. Daddy and I are so proud of our little trooper.

Sofia is now on 3 milliliters an hour of my milk, and she certainly loves it!

February 23—Ten days old

Oh my God!! Our little girl seems bigger today! Sofia's skin appears more baby-like and she seems to be filling out.

Sofia is now on 4.2 milliliters an hour of feed (milk), which is the maximum amount for her weight of 1.5 pounds.

She is still not ready to come off the ventilator, maybe tomorrow.

Daddy fed Sofia twice tonight while I went off to the milking cupboard.

February 24—Eleven days old

Baby Sofia is back on CPAP. She needed another blood transfusion today and a change of cannula (a little tube inserted into one of the veins in her body to administer medication and fluids).

Poppet seemed quieter today, possibly because she has been through a lot in one day. Daddy and I felt that Little One was too tired and had been disturbed too much for one day.

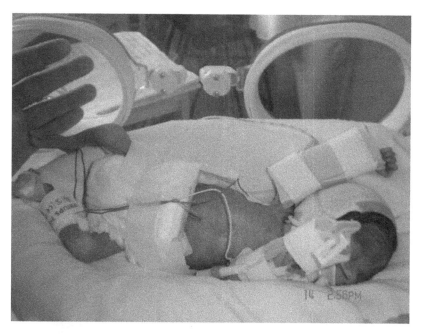

Sofia and her surfboards. As you can see, Sofia's skin has lost that waxy appearance.

Daddy gave Sofia another baby bed bath and changed a very dirty nappy and both of us carried out Sofia's feedings.

Granddad Vercesi filmed Daddy feeding Sofia, and Daddy took some more pictures for the family album. Again off I went to the milking cupboard.

February 25—Twelve days old

Today was a very big day for our little family. Daddy and I went to register Sofia's birth. We then headed straight to the hospital to see our beautiful little girl and to officially change her name from Baby Meechan to Baby Vercesi on all her medical records.

The most incredible part of this day occurred when we held our precious tiny bundle in our arms for the very first time. I cried yet again—what a wuss! It was the most amazing moment after the birth of Sofia to finally hold her close to us. Little Poppet seemed to know that she was in our arms too as she snuggled down like a little bug in a rug. It was both wonderful and extraordinary, the three of us in our own little world. I couldn't believe just how light she felt and how tiny she was outside her little greenhouse. Sofia was wrapped in lots of blankets to make sure her temperature didn't drop.

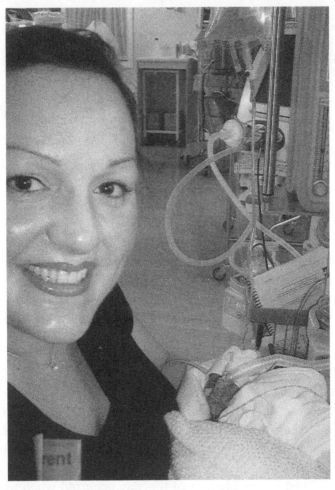

The very first time I held my baby, and I was the happiest woman in the world. I couldn't help but sob tears of joy. Sofia's tiny head is just about visible. The CPAP is attached to help with her breathing.

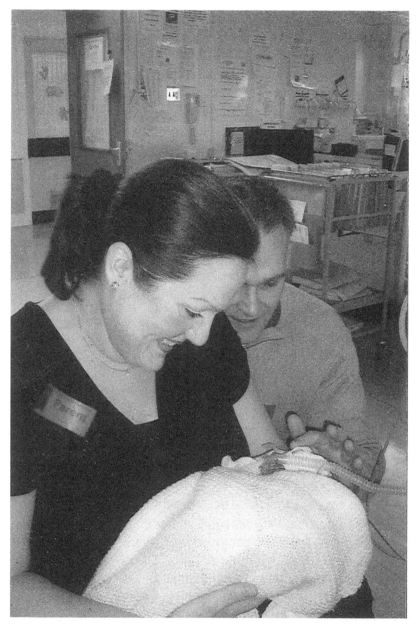

Our little family having our very first cuddle together. Sofia is wrapped in many layers of blankets to help maintain her body temperature.

Later in the evening I tried to do Sofia's baby bed bath. I was completely hopeless and couldn't get anything right; even the nappy change floored me! I had a little cry at this.

It's official! Our daughter is a mini pooping machine. What a dirty bottom! It was everywhere. Again I didn't do too well so Daddy had to take over. I just get too frightened. Then to top it off, Sofia launched a little missile poo from that wrinkly bottom and it hit the end of the incubator. Daddy laughed his socks off at this; he was impressed.

Our baby girl has lost weight today. Not good.

Daddy and I just can't wait to take our baby home. Daddy was sure he could even fit Sofia in his pocket and smuggle her out.

Overall, today was a very big day for our little family. Words cannot describe how amazing it was to finally hold our very special angel.

February 26—Thirteen days old

Yet again, Poppet has lost weight and she is now weighing 1.3 pounds. The doctors think that Sofia is not getting enough nutrients so they are going to add them to my milk.

Sofia now has both eyes open and she seems to watch Daddy and me. Well, that's what we blissfully believe she is doing.

Daddy and I shared baby bed bath time today. I did Sofia's face while Daddy dealt with Poppet's sore little bottom. Our little pooping machine decided to poop all over Daddy's finger. Oops! I had a giggle at this.

Sofia now has to have special cream applied to her bottom. It has become very, very sore due to her poops being so runny.

Tonight we left Sofia snuggled up with a special blanket that I had knitted and worn against my skin. The purpose of this is to enable Sofia to smell me. After leaving it inside Sofia's incubator I then take the blanket and wear it against my skin in attempt to encourage my milk flow as I smell my baby's scent. Again, to me this is a gift. It is what mothers take for granted, and quite rightly so. But for me being able to smell my baby's scent I have to leave items inside her incubator and hope that they will hold my daughter's smell, and more importantly enable Sofia to recognise her mommy's smell too. I am terrified that she will not even know her own mommy.

Two Weeks Old

February 27—Fourteen days old

Baby Sofia is two weeks old today.

Today was Mommy and Baby Day. Daddy had to go to Uncle Wayne's funeral in Wales. Uncle Wayne never got to meet Sofia; he died tragically four days after her birth.

Sofia and I chilled out and did girly things today. That is, I sat at Poppet's bedside and talked to her through the incubator and stroked her little head.

Little Sofia is now weighing 1.4 pounds.

Tonight when I carried out Sofia's baby bed bath I found that she had left a tiny poo in her nappy for me.

She cried a bit today. Being moved and handled visibly distressed her, and she also seemed very uncomfortable. She soon calmed down when I stroked her tiny body; I think she knows that her mommy is touching her.

February 28—Fifteen days old

Little Sofia is poorly today. She had a bad night with a number of desat episodes. A desat is when the amount of oxygen in the blood decreases. Basically this means that Little One has less oxygen than her body needs to cope. It is important that the right balance is made when administering oxygen because too much can damage the baby's eyes and too little can make the baby very unwell. If the baby stops breathing for more than fifteen to twenty seconds then a situation known as apnoea occurs. It tends to go hand in hand with a bradycardia. A bradycardia, or brady as we know it, is when the heart slows right down. During this the baby will develop a bluish tinge to her lips and exhibit a pale, blotchy skin colour (mottled) and then become quite limp. This can be very bad, and if the baby's heart rate does not recover then rigorous stimulation will be needed before they try and "bag" the baby, meaning they carry out "baby CPR" to restimulate her little heart and brain. This situation requires immediate attention because if left the baby can die.

When Daddy and I arrived at the hospital today Sofia was back on the ventilator again; she is simply struggling to cope on her own.

Sofia had to have another chest X-ray and it showed that not only do her lungs appear to be collapsing but they are also full of fluid. Sofia has now started having physiotherapy (physio) to try and loosen the secretions in her lungs, which act like glue, so every time Sofia breathes out her lungs stick together and struggle to open back up when she breathes in. The physio involves her having vigorous tapping all around her chest and then a tube is inserted into her mouth to suction and remove the excess fluid that has been loosened and dislodged. It is difficult to witness this procedure as a parent, watching your tiny baby receiving such aggressive physio. At first I had to stop myself from jumping on the nurse's back and telling her to leave my baby alone. Even though I knew it was a vital procedure, it just seemed so barbaric. But considering everything Sofia has had to endure it was yet another necessary procedure required to keep my baby alive.

Poppet still has a heart murmur and she has been put onto medication (Indomethacin) for six days to see if it will close the duct in her heart that is causing the murmur. Unfortunately when babies are born as early as Poppet a duct in their hearts can fail to close after birth. This is known as Patent Ductus Arteriosus (PDA). In healthy, full-term births this duct begins to close over once the baby takes her first breath and within a few weeks it has fully closed. However, in Sofia's case this duct was showing no signs of closing, hence the need to use the drug Indomethacin. If necessary this injection is normally given within the first two weeks of a baby's life. If this treatment fails then Sofia will need surgery on her tiny little heart.

Sofia has been put back on antibiotics and is now nil by mouth, with her receiving nutrients via a drip (dextrose).

Sofia's tummy was very swollen tonight and the doctors had to examine her. They may need to take another X-ray.

Poppet's little poops are yellow at the moment.

Sofia was very quiet tonight and she didn't even manage to open her eyes for Daddy and me.

Little One's blood gases are ok. This is a test carried out on the blood to check that it contains the correct amount of oxygen or carbon dioxide and if the blood has the right acid balance. From this test the doctors are able to monitor the baby's respiratory status as well as a number of other functions that rely on the use of energy production performed within the body. This is one of the tests that have to be performed frequently. Unfortunately it is also a test that yet again involves taking vital blood from our baby's body.

March 1—Sixteen days old (27th week of gestation)

Sofia is still a very poorly little girl today. She is now on antibiotics for her tummy and lungs and she is on morphine for pain and dextrose (for her nutrients).

Sofia's little tummy is not so distended today and it seems to be gradually reducing in size. Poppet continues to remain nil by mouth and she's still on the life support ventilator.

Sofia's urine output is poor so they have had to stop her heart medication for the time being.

Sofia also had to have part of a gelatine capsule put into her bottom to try and help her poop.

Little One has green bile in her tummy. Again the doctors and nurses informed us that these are all frequently observed complications with little people who are born as early as our little princess.

On the bright side, Sofia seems more stable and is opening her eyes and squeezing the tips of our fingers. Then the little rascal had the biggest tiny temper tantrum and those little arms and legs were all over the place.

March 2—Seventeen days old

Sofia has been stable today. However, she is still on all her antibiotics, dextrose, morphine, and other medications. Her tummy has also continued to reduce in size.

Poppet is now passing water again and I was so happy to change a wet nappy tonight. Today Sofia had a heart scan to monitor the duct. The doctor performed the scan while I was with Sofia. Unfortunately the duct has not closed and it looks like our little girl will undergo heart surgery when she recovers from her staphylococcus infection (bacterial infection). Plus it looks like the Indomethacin injection caused Sofia kidney problems, which is why her urine output ceased and Sofia went into renal failure. Because of this, it seems highly unlikely that she will have any more of that injection.

Poppet is still nil by mouth. She managed a little poop last night, which is good news.

Little One's weight was 1.5 pounds today; however, we are not sure how much of this is due to the ventilator pipe in her lungs.

We are still trying to work out who Sofia looks like. I want to put little bows in her hair. She is a very beautiful little girl. I think Sofia has Daddy's nose and camel eye lashes. Sofia definitely has Daddy's long legs.

Sofia's little bottom doesn't look so sore tonight, which is good. It really upsets Daddy and me knowing that our tiny bundle is in pain and suffering.

A certain young lady managed to pull her nasal gastric tube from her nose tonight and Daddy had to pry it from Sofia's tiny little fingers.

March 3—Eighteen days old

Little Sofia gets more and more beautiful with each passing day.

When Daddy and I arrived today Sofia had just been moved back on to CPAP, which is fantastic news.

The bug Sofia has been fighting has now been identified and treated with yet another antibiotic.

I became upset today because our baby girl had a lumbar puncture (this is when a needle is inserted into the space in the lower part of the spine and used to withdraw spinal fluid for testing) to see if her infection has affected her brain, such as meningitis. Sofia also had a needle inserted into her bladder to try and draw out urine. The needle inserted into Sofia's bladder didn't work, but luckily the lumbar puncture came back negative.

Poppet is now back on my milk. She started off on low quantities of feed but will return to 4.2 milliliters an hour overnight.

There is still no news on Sofia's heart; we will have to wait till the infection has gone to see if it caused the duct to open.

Daddy and I miss Poppet so much when we are not with her and we keep praying that our little girl will get stronger and become a chubby little monkey on my milk, so Mommy and Daddy can take her home.

March 4—Nineteen days old

Today was a really big day in Sofia's life. She is steadily recovering from her infection and will remain on antibiotics for the next ten to twelve days. We are still unsure about the heart surgery because this is dependent on whether the infection is responsible for the duct remaining open.

The best news of the day, albeit a little scary, is that little Sofia has been moved to a new room. She's still in a high dependency room, but this is one where she is considered stable enough to be in.

Poppet is also able to breathe a little better today too.

One of Sofia's little roommates is extremely poorly, which meant we were unable to spend a great deal of time with her today.

March 5—Twenty days old

Poppet is struggling with her breathing again. She keeps having desats.

Another heart scan revealed the duct has opened more and now blood is gushing through it willy nilly. But we are still waiting for the infection to come under control. They are reducing Little One's fluid intake and giving her diuretics (substances used to increase the amount of urine produced) to reduce the strain on her heart and they have also increased her oxygen levels. It looks like heart surgery is definitely in the cards.

Our baby is so beautiful and we just want her to get better and bigger and stronger.

Poppet also has a small amount of blood in her urine, but we are not sure of the cause yet. It is possibly from the test they carried out the other day when they stuck a needle into her bladder.

Three Weeks Old

March 6—Twenty-one days old

Poppet is three weeks old today.

Little One had a couple of desats again overnight and her skin seems pale.

Daddy and I held Sofia again today and it was amazing. It's as though she knows it's us and just calms right down. Our tiny little bundle snuggles in our arms and watches us. Heaven.

Daddy filmed Sofia and I, and then I filmed Daddy and Sofia.

Daddy did the baby bed bath today.

We tucked Little One up for the night in her little greenhouse and made sure she was asleep before we left her.

March 7—Twenty-two days old

Little One had a more stable night. However, her colour is still quite "mottled" (this is when the skin appears to be like marble) and she seems quite tired today.

Both Daddy and I held Sofia today and she seemed to enjoy it.

They are still not able to find a happy medium with Little One's oxygen.

The nurse practitioner (this is an individual with advanced nursing qualifications enabling them to perform more specialised techniques) had problems trying to get Little One's blood tonight. Sofia's veins are as thin as a strand of hair and extremely fragile and difficult to work with, especially because all the accessible ones have already been used and are in the process of healing. She told us she had forgotten just how tiny Sofia is. She's our little Polly Pocket.

Poppet is going to have a drip again because she has passed very little urine.

The more we hold Poppet the more we want to bring her home. It is the most magical feeling in the world to hold your child close to you. I cannot wait for skin to skin contact. Skin to skin is exactly what it says. It is when you hold your baby against your bare flesh. It is a beautiful bonding experience for the baby and parent, and in the case of the mother it is also another way of helping stimulate milk flow.

March 8—Twenty-three days old (28th week of gestation)

Sofia's skin is still very pale. She is still on a drip while they try to re-hydrate her little body.

Sofia and I had our first skin to skin contact today and it was the loveliest feeling in the world. We were both blissfully content. Little One snuggled right into me. I just didn't want it to end, the feeling of those gentle little flutters of movement from her teeny limbs. It's strange to imagine that this is a sensation I should be experiencing from inside my tummy.

I changed a very dirty nappy tonight and the little monkey has now learned to stretch her legs out to make it difficult. She certainly likes to play games, the little rascal.

Poppet's weight has gone up slightly and her feedings are now at 4.2 milliliters an hour.

Sofia made Daddy laugh today because it looked like she was waving to him.

March 9—Twenty-four days old

Today has been a very hard day for our little precious. After an awful night full of desats and brady cardy attacks, Little One had to be put back on to the life support ventilator. She is just so weak at the moment.

Another blood transfusion was carried out in the early hours of the morning, and now Poppet is nice and pink again.

Sofia is still not having any luck with fighting her infection. The doctors have changed her antibiotics again. She is still having problems with her kidney function too. Her urine output is very poor.

Talks have been had with a specialist children's hospital regarding Sofia's heart surgery, which they now consider a necessity. However, this cannot be performed until the infection has been dealt with, because Sofia is just so vulnerable and weak. She needs all the strength that she can muster when she undergoes her heart surgery.

Tonight Poppet vomited so her feedings have been stopped till 2 a.m. Her tummy is still very bloated and she has had to have another suppository. She may need another abdominal X-ray if things don't change.

Sofia's breathing and heart rate appear more settled for now.

It has been a very stressful day today; our little fighter has to work so hard to stay alive.

March 10—Twenty-five days old

Sofia is still very ill. She had another desat this morning but this might have been caused by her neck bending.

Poppet has had a second lumbar puncture and another blood transfusion today.

They are now weaning her off one antibiotic on to another, which hopefully will be less damaging to her kidneys. She is still in renal failure, which could be due to the medication because her kidneys are just not developed enough to cope.

Poppet's temperature is up and down and she is still nil by mouth, although tonight they are going to resume her feeding in small quantities.

Little One seemed to be more alert today and she was awake most of the time. We witnessed a number of little temper tantrums, which we are finding both funny and painful to watch because both her frustration and discomfort are obvious.

Sofia held mine and Daddy's little fingers tightly tonight, which we absolutely loved. We don't want to ever let her go.

Poppet's weight is at 1.6 pounds, but this may be due to the water retention.

March 11—Twenty-six days old

Little One is more alert today.

Sofia's heart surgery was originally booked for 10 a.m. on March 12 so Daddy and I had asked for a priest to attend the unit to Baptise our little angel. The specialist children's hospital then called and changed the date of Sofia's surgery to March 13 (yet again another Friday the 13th!). The priest arrived at the hospital this evening and conducted a very touching service. Grandma and Granddad Vercesi also came to the hospital to be present for the ceremony. Baby Sofia wore a beautiful knitted pink bat cape with little roses stitched on. Our mini crusader. Partway through the service Sofia shocked us all. All of a sudden those beautiful little eyes opened and the readings on her life support machine seemed to stabilise. Sofia was breathing all on her own without any help from the machine. Even the priest noticed and commented that we have a very special little girl. It felt very spiritual, and we honestly felt as though Sofia was being watched over and protected and that she also knew exactly what was going on.

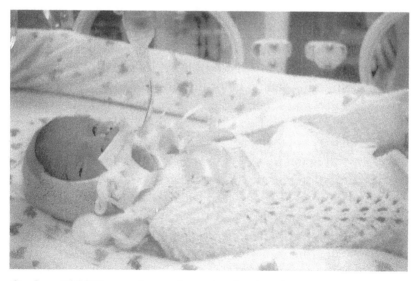

Our beautiful little caped crusader on her baptism day

Little One frightened me earlier in the evening when I changed her nappy. Poppet decided that she was going to have a desat. Apparently this is one of her little tricks when being handled. I was a nervous wreck. She was grounded for that.

Today was a very wriggly day today for our beautiful little girl.

March 12—Twenty-seven days old

Day before the heart surgery.

Little One is quite stable today and settled. Her weight has dropped again, but this could be due to the retained water.

I spent most of the day at Sofia's bedside, too afraid of what was to come. Cannot write much today. It is the not knowing. I am struggling to be brave.

Four Weeks Old

March 13—Twenty-eight days old

Darn Friday the 13th again!

Poppet is one month old today, and it is big heart surgery day.

Daddy went to Sofia's normal hospital while I went to the specialist children's hospital to be with Poppet on her arrival. I wasn't able to travel with Poppet because she was transported on a life support machine, which in itself could kill her. Yet again another worry, but this is the only way Sofia will live. I had to rely on both trains and taxis for the day.

I was a nervous wreck while I waited for my baby to arrive at the children's hospital. I was so happy that Little One had made the first journey but then I couldn't help but become upset that my tiny baby was about to undergo surgery, which could kill her too.

There was a problem with the paperwork that came over with Sofia's bags of blood, so the hospital ended up rejecting the blood. This resulted in both Sofia and I having to give blood for cross-referencing in case Little One needed a blood transfusion while in the operating theatre. This made me very angry because I was told that this is a regular problem faced by the hospital and to date nobody has sought to resolve it. Not only were valuable bags of blood destroyed because the paperwork was unacceptable but Sofia had to give blood again, of which she had very little. It certainly didn't give me much confidence in what she was about to undergo.

A special type of 4D heart scan was carried out on Sofia prior to the surgery, and the specialist informed me that they had to perform this to see if she had any other heart complications that have not been detected yet, as they could potentially kill her if undetected or they could mean that the surgery she was about to undergo was unnecessary because her heart would not improve. Thank God the scan came back as confirmation that she had just the one problem.

The strangest phenomenon occurred as they performed the scan. A magical connection between Sofia and I seemed to happen that only we understood. Sofia seemed to look straight into my eyes and she held on so tight to my little fingertip and then squeezed me as hard as those little fingers could manage. I was trying desperately hard not to sob as they were about to take my precious baby away. It was as though Sofia was telling me to be strong and that she would be okay. Those little eyes never once left my face. It comes to something when your tiny bundle is the one demonstrating tremendous strength and courage.

Because Sofia is so tiny, they are using specialist microscopic equipment to perform the surgery on her heart. They will also have to access her heart through the side of her rib cage. The consultant informed me that there is a slight possibility of Sofia developing a slight dip in posture on the left side due to this intervention, but to be honest I really didn't give a damn; I just wanted my beautiful baby to be kept alive.

At 11 a.m. Sofia was wheeled away from me and taken into the operating theatre. It was the hardest thing I have ever had to do, to sit and watch as they took my baby from me. I broke down and sobbed, and prayed to God to please keep her safe. Don't take my baby. I felt so helpless.

The operation itself took about an hour and a half, and I was the happiest woman in the world when my precious angel was wheeled back to me. Thank you, God. The surgery had been successful and Sofia now has a tiny clip in her heart.

Looks like Poppet left her mark at the specialist children's hospital, as she left lots of poop and pee on the operating table.

That's my girl. Sofia was stabilised on the travel life support machine before being prepared for the return journey. I set back off for the train station while Poppet was traveling by her preferred method of ambulance.

Poppet made the return journey successfully and is now settled and as high as a kite on morphine and away with the fairies. Again, thank God for her safe return.

Daddy and I left the hospital early in the evening to let our precious angel rest. Thanks to the incredible skills of a fantastic surgeon, Sofia now has a tiny metal clip in her heart, which, knock on wood, will work.

March 14—Twenty-nine days old

Poppet is stable. She's still a little groggy with her morphine and she is still having desats and bradys when being handled.

We have a very sleepy little girl today.

Sofia managed to hold on to our fingers a little and even managed to open her eyes a couple of times today.

Over the day Little One gradually had her milk reintroduced, starting with 1 milliliter an hour.

We are certain our little caped crusader has grown. Sofia's little tiny fingers look like they are a little chubbier, little micro sausages. Poppet also tends to bend her toes upward just like I do; we expect to find lots of mini shoes with curled up toe areas when she comes home. Our little girl was scrunched up like a little diddy frog today.

Daddy was like David Bailey with the camera.

March 15—Thirty days old (29th week of gestation)

Little One looked so lovely and peaceful today; she seems a lot more comfortable.

They have now begun weaning Poppet today for extubation, which is the removal of the life support tube from Poppet for her to go back onto CPAP. Poppet is now off the morphine. Our incredibly brave little girl.

Handling seems to be a bit less stressful for our angel and her blood gases are looking good so it looks like her little body is coping.

Poppet had yet another blood transfusion today.

March 16—Thirty-one days old

Sofia is back on CPAP today. She is also on 3 milliliters an hour feedings and she now weighs a whopping 1.63 pounds. Her biggest weight yet!

I had a beautiful little cuddle today with my girl.

Poppet is still very sore and it shows in her respiratory rate. Those lovely little eyes had a peep a few times. Sneaky.

March 17—Thirty-two days old

Little One is progressing steadily.

Today was a big day for Poppet. Not only did she show off her gorgeous Mohican hairstyle but most importantly she had an hour in her little incubator without any breathing assistance. I didn't recognise my little girl today because I'd never seen her before without her special hats on. She looked like a beautiful little pocket-sized werewolf, a werebaby.

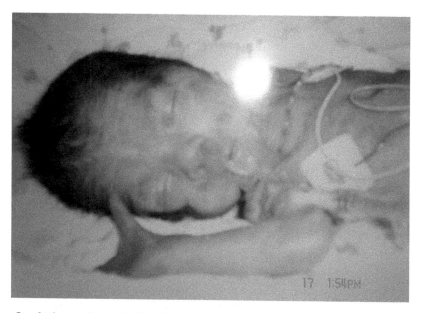

Our little werebaby. Sofia's face is covered in sores and creases where her masks have dented her chops.

Sofia's feedings are now up to 4.5 milliliters an hour.

Little Poppet also wore a little pink vest today and she looked absolutely beautiful.

I had another snuggle today and even kissed her on the cheek for the very first time. The nurse let me do it.

Poppet will have another hour off the oxygen tonight.

March 18—Thirty-three days old

Little One is stable and still having an hour off her masks (oxygen). She is now on 5 milliliters (a teaspoon) an hour and her weight is at 1.5 pounds.

We had another snuggle today and Poppet even snuggled under my top. I think she was planning her escape.

Sofia is now off the antibiotics but she still has a tiny heart murmur.

March 19—Thirty-four days old

Little One is now back in the second intensive care room, therefore she has less supervision again.

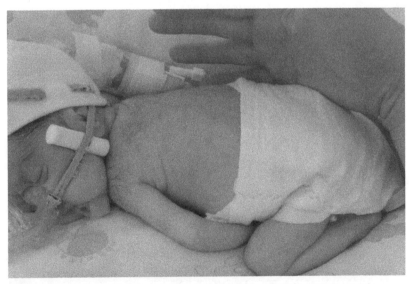

Nanny and Granddad (Mom and John) took this picture of Sofia, and you can just about make out the scar left by the heart surgery over her ribs. She is also extremely pale due to her anaemia.

Sofia is still 1.5 pounds and she still on 5 milliliters of milk an hour with added fortifier. Daddy and I each did some feedings today.

I had a really big snuggle today with Sofia, which really cheered me up. Little One doesn't seem to like going back into the incubator after snuggling. Daddy and I hate her having to go back into it too.

Our little angel looks more and more beautiful each day and she makes the loveliest noises in the world.

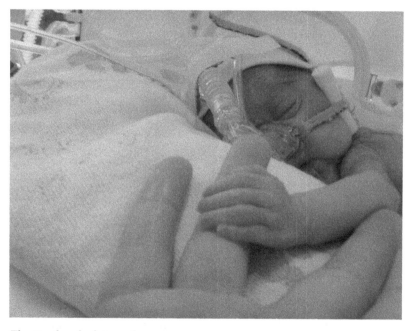

The tiny hand of strength

Five Weeks Old

March 20—Thirty-five days old

Sofia is five weeks old today and she looked absolutely beautiful in a little dolls flower dress. Very *Little House on the Prairie.*

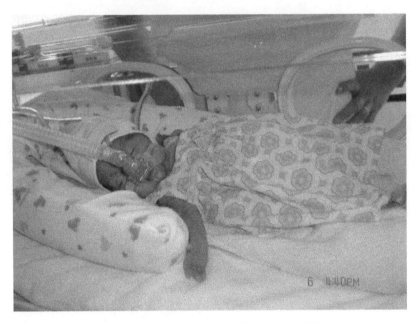

Poppet in her Little House on the Prairie *dolls dress on CPAP*

Sofia is now on 6 milliliters of feeding an hour and weighing in at 1.6 pounds.

Sofia has been moved to room 1 with even less supervision. She is now on normal CPAP (NCPAP). However, if Poppet's blood gases don't improve then she will go back on to biphasic CPAP (this gives the baby more help than the NCPAP and maintains a safe pressure in their lungs). Hopefully this will do enough to keep her off the life support ventilator.

No cuddles today due to Sofia's change in breathing support. It's best she's not too stressed, as it will tire her little body out.

March 21—Thirty-six days old

Little Sofia is definitely more and more beautiful with each passing day. Today it looks like our little girl is trying to smile. Gorgeous!!!

Unfortunately Poppet has gone back onto biphasic CPAP. Too much too soon. Her breathing is not brilliant. She is still up and down with desats, but Poppet is so tiny she needs more time.

50

Sofia now weighs 1.61 pounds and she is still on 6-milliliter hourly feeds.

Poppet watched me today as I changed her smelly little nappy and my clever little girl did a poo and lots of wee, which is what we like to see.

March 22—Thirty-seven days old (30th week of gestation)

Our first Mother's Day!

It was a sad start to the day because Poppet has been having a lot of desats and bradys. They think it may be caused by the feed refluxing, so Gaviscon has been added to thicken up the feeds and weigh them down.

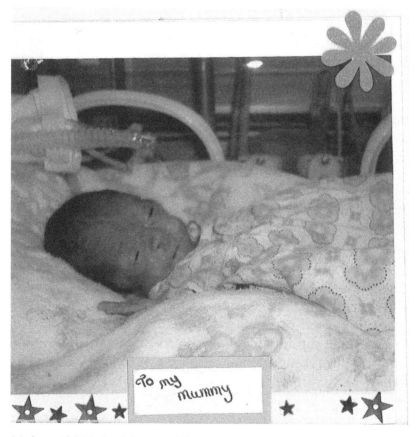

My beautiful Mother's Day card from a very poor-looking Sofia dressed in a dolls dress

The nurses have made me a wonderful card with a picture of our beautiful little girl in a little frock. I was also given a box of chocolates. This really made my day.

Poppet was fairly stable during the afternoon but she was a cheeky little monkey when Daddy did her baby bed bath. Somehow, our little rascal, while wide awake, kept managing to set off her alarms while looking very wide-eyed and innocent at both Daddy and I.

Aunty Nus and Aunty Finola came to see me at home today before I left for the hospital and they were loaded with gifts from the team at work.

March 23—Thirty-eight days old

Little One is still poorly, very much the same as yesterday with lots of desats and bradys.

Sofia now weighs a massive 1.7 pounds!

The doctors have started Poppet on antibiotics again.

I had another skin to skin cuddle today and Poppet kept nudging my chest with her tiny little head. Daddy had a snuggle with his little Poppet too. Sofia seems to like watching while she has her bottom changed. I even managed to do Sofia's baby bed bath today.

March 24—Thirty-nine days old

Sofia is still a poorly girl. She has been having lots of desats and stuff.

Poppet is now weighing a whopping 1.83 pounds, our little chunky monkey. Our little monkey is certainly growing. It's just heartbreaking that she is poorly again.

Sofia's blood gases are relatively okay although there has been a slight dip in her haemoglobin (Hb) level. It has gone from 13 to 11. Haemoglobin is present in red blood cells and its function is to carry oxygen to the rest of the body. I understand that the range for children is between 11 to 16 G/dL (grams per deciliter). Sofia's is still within range at the moment, but if it continues to drop then she will begin to struggle again.

Sofia has a slightly raised CRP (C Reactive Protein). This is a chemical found in the body that increases in response to bacterial and viral infections among other medical conditions. I understand that if the CRP level is in excess of 3.0 mg/L then it is considered to be high, and greater than 10 indicates severe infection. Sofia was showing signs of yet another infection again.

Because Sofia is a little rascal, the doctors think that she is losing air through her mouth because our little girl has a tendency to catch flies all day. Today, the nurses have wedged a roll of gauze under her little chin. Now Sofia looks like a tiny chipmunk with those chubby chops.

Daddy and I both had skin to skin cuddles with Poppet.

I did Sofia's baby bed bath today. I'm still a nervous wreck.

Sofia's X-rays are showing patches of white on her lungs, which is not a good sign at all.

March 25—Forty days old

Poppet is still very poorly and she has been having lots of desats and bradys.

Sofia was started on diuretics again today.

I am happy to report that I changed a very dirty nappy.

Sofia and I had a little snuggle today. Sofia keeps suckling but her tiny little mouth is too small even for the smallest of dummies.

Sofia's weight is still at 1.8 pounds.

March 26—Forty-one days old

A very bad day. I was phoned just after 4 a.m. by one of the nurses. Our precious baby had stopped breathing. It took eight minutes for the doctors and nurses to bring Sofia back ("bag"). Daddy and I went straight to the hospital and Little One had to be put back on to the life support machine again. It took hours before Sofia was stabilised again.

Daddy and I have been told that Sofia is very, very ill, and she is not responding to treatment. It looks like she needs a steroid called Dexamethasone. This drug is used as an anti-inflammatory medication to try and help the lungs work. Sofia has so much fluid on her underdeveloped lungs that they simply cannot work. The drug is associated with developmental problems such as cerebral palsy, and because of this permission has to be given by the parents before it is administered. We were told that this is a last resort and it's not even guaranteed to work. Therefore if we choose not to let Sofia have the drug then she will inevitably pass away. So no matter what choice you make you are being asked to play God with your child's life. A devastating blow to Daddy and I. I would give up my life to save my beautiful baby daughter! I broke down at this news and the nurses took Sofia out of her incubator and put her into my arms. I held her so tight. It was so scary for me because I've never held Sofia before when she was on life support and I was so frightened I might hurt her. But the nurse's taped Sofia's breathing tubes to my arms. Daddy and I stroked Sofia and kept telling her how much we love her and that she's got to keep fighting.

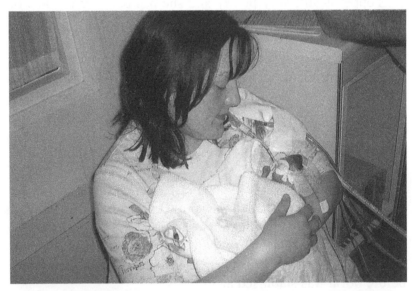

The day after Sofia was "bagged" for eight minutes and we were told to expect the worst. Sofia's life support tube is taped to my shoulder. This news was incredibly hard for me to handle and I couldn't stop my tears.

Six Weeks Old

March 27—Forty-two days old

Sofia is fairly stable today, but far from brilliant!

Poppet is not responding to the diuretics. It is very hard for Daddy and me because when our darling is awake she becomes very distressed and she absolutely hates being handled at the moment. We feel so unbelievably helpless.

Daddy and I have been having very long talks with the doctors.

March 28—Forty-three days old

Sofia is still no better today and she still needs lots of suction.

Poppet's feedings have now gone up to 4 milliliters an hour.

Sofia's sats are not good and the CRP test has shown yet another bug, which now has to be treated before the steroids can be started.

I am now finding it all too much, and ashamedly I keep breaking down.

I DON'T WANT TO LOSE MY BABY!!!

Sofia is so stunningly beautiful and she needs all the help and prayers she can get. We keep praying that our beautiful angel will get better.

I had a lovely snuggle today with my baby and I cherished the feeling of holding her close to my body.

March 29—Forty-four days old (31st week of gestation)

Poppet is more stable today.

Sofia definitely has a little temper, which is very apparent. Even when she is tucked up in her incubator she likes to be involved in a conversation, and if not, boy, does she have a little rant, which affects her settings, resulting in beeps and alarms going off left, right, and centre.

Those beautiful little eyes keep watching everybody, and I am convinced they are going to be brown. Daddy keeps saying they are going to be blue. Mind you, Daddy was convinced we were going to have a little boy. So I remind of him of this every now and again just to be cheeky.

I had a lovely cuddle with Sofia and Little One seemed to love it too.

Daddy did Sofia's baby bed bath today. He chats away to his little girl and I'm sure she's taking it all in.

March 30—Forty-five days old

Little One had a stable night and day and even had a skin to skin cuddle with me. Sofia likes to peep at me when she thinks that I'm not watching and then when I look at her she quickly closes her eyes. The little sneaky monkey.

Today I did Sofia's baby bed bath and one of the nurses put some of my milk on a sterile cotton bud for Sofia to suck. Little One loved it and wouldn't let me have the bud back. It was the very first time Sofia had actually tasted my milk because the feeding tubes have always prevented it before.

March 31—Forty-six days old

Fantastic news! Sofia has been so good that the doctors have decided it would be better to extubate her back on to CPAP. This means she may not need the steroid. YIPEEEEEEEEE!!! I could cry. When I arrived at the unit Little One had only just been changed back over on to less support.

Sofia's CRP level is now at 4, which is not brilliant but not as bad as it has been.

I am very scared and worried that Sofia will have a repeat of last week, knowing just how quickly she can deteriorate.

Poppet seems happier now that she has had that tube taken out of her lungs. Yet again someone up there seems to be watching over our precious little girl.

April 1—Forty-seven days old

Little One is still nice and stable, knock on wood.

Sofia's weight has dropped to 1.9 pounds again. She is very sleepy today.

Sofia had her first eye screening today, as they need to check for abnormalities, which apparently are common among babies born so prematurely. The eye specialist was happy today, but he now needs to check each week because it is still early. Yet again, this is something else to worry about. They are testing for a condition known as ROP (Retinopathy of Prematurity), which is basically when blood vessels grow like weeds over the retinas and if left untreated will result in blindness. This is sadly yet another consequence of being born so premature.

April 2—Forty-eight days old

Little One is fine again today; she has had a couple of bradys and desats, though.

I had a snuggle with Poppet today but Daddy couldn't because he has got man flu.

Sofia is back to 6-milliliter-an-hour feedings.

Seven Weeks Old

April 3—Forty-nine days old

Sofia is fairly stable today. Her weight is now approximately 2 pounds and she is now on 6.5 milliliter feedings an hour.

Today was absolutely amazing for Sofia and me. Tiny Sofia suckled from me a little bit today and made me the happiest mommy in the world.

Sofia decided to poo on me at baby bed bath time, which was very funny indeed. She's such a little monkey.

Poppet is still looking a bit pale, and she definitely hates the suction of her secretions. Who wouldn't?

April 4—Fifty days old

Sofia is 1.8 pounds today.

Poppet really scared Daddy and me today. She had a massive desat and brady, and Daddy had to go and call the nurse because no one came when the alarms were set off. Little One later calmed down, but she still continued to have a few little desats.

Sofia still needs loads of suction and her Hb is 12.8.

Poppet had a fight with the nurse over her nasal prongs and Poppet won round 1 but the nurse won round 2. Sofia absolutely detests nasal prongs.

April 5—Fifty-one days old (32nd week of gestation)

Sofia's weight is 1.9 pounds today.

Little One has been having clusters of desats and bradys and her Hb is now 11.7. It is dropping again.

Sofia and I had a little snuggle, which was brilliant. Poppet hates going back into her den after snuggles and she isn't afraid to show it via a desat!

Daddy and I know how Little One works now. Sofia is quite happy during baby bed bath time and she loves cuddle time. What she absolutely hates is a dirty bottom, being on the ventilator, being put back into her tub, and those horrid nasal prongs.

Sofia is now on to two hourly suctions.

Sofia and I were colour-coordinated today and we both wore pink and white outfits.

April 6—Fifty-two days old

Little One is now weighing 2 pounds. Wow!

Sofia and I had another wonderful snuggle today.

She is fairly stable and those big, wide eyes were very alert in the evening. The little hamster.

April 7—Fifty-three days old

Little One is now at 2 pounds and off CPAP.

Sofia was very pale and cold when I arrived at the hospital so no cuddles today. Her Hb is at 12.

Sofia frightened me tonight when the doctors were doing their ward rounds. She had a very bad desat and brady. The doctors had to use "Tom Thumb." It is a piece of medical equipment used for resuscitation. Not good. Not good at all. When Sofia was stabilised she needed suction again and a big plug of thick, white secretion was removed from her throat. Afterward Little One had a chest X-ray and it showed "foggy" patches on the right side of her lungs. The doctors told us that Sofia needs physio and medication again.

Daddy and I are very worried!

April 8—Fifty-four days old

Sofia is fairly stable today. She is now on continuous feedings instead of hourly feeds. This is to try and stop the refluxing (this is basically when Sofia's milk backflows against the normal flow so instead of staying in the stomach the milk comes out and back up). This method of feeding involves the milk being put into a syringe driver and slowly trickled into her tummy continuously. Apparently using this technique reduces the chance of reflux, which in turn should reduce desats.

Sofia's weight has dropped again and now she is back at 1.9 pounds.

Little One had another eye test again today and it went well. Fingers crossed.

Yet another blood transfusion is planned for later because Sofia's Hb has dropped to 9, which is very low.

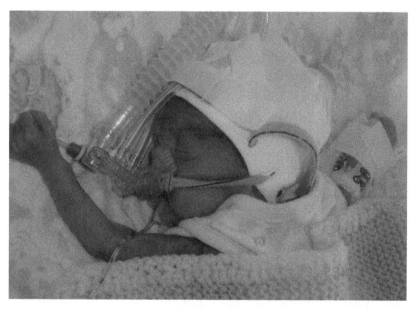

Sofia wearing her special hat with the CPAP attached

I was able to do the baby bed bath today. Little tufts of black hair are now popping out through the back of Sofia's surgical bonnet. Babies as small as Sofia wear special bonnets that are designed specifically to help hold the ventilator tubes in place. I tried to put teeny mittens on Poppet today, but because her hands are so incredibly tiny, as soon as she moves they fly off and I had to keep rummaging inside her incubator to try and find them.

April 9—Fifty-five days old

Little One is fairly stable again, although she still has loads of rubbish in her throat, which is having to be suctioned out.

Sofia's weight has increased a little today and she is now 1.9 pounds.

I carried out Sofia's baby bed bath again today and I even managed to put a little sleep suit on her. This was very hard for me because Sofia is so tiny and fragile and I am so frightened of hurting her.

Poppet's feed is now up to 8 milliliters continuously. We need to make her bigger. She is just so tiny.

Sofia had her beautiful, big eyes open a bit today and they are starting to look a bit blue. Sofia also has the most beautiful head of dark hair.

Somehow a certain young lady has lost one of her mittens. I am perplexed; she lives in a tiny little box and nothing can get in or out without opening the doors. It's puzzling.

Eight Weeks Old

April 10—Fifty-six days old

Sofia is now a whopping 2.1 pounds today (although some of it will be CPAP). My little chunky monkey.

I carried out Little One's baby bed bath today. Daddy came to the unit later in the day.

Yet again I saw my beautiful girl's head of hair and those enormous eyes, which watched me as I pottered around the outside of her incubator. I couldn't stop giggling at Sofia today; she kept moving her little head to spy on me.

April 11—Fifty-seven days old

Little One has dropped to 2 pounds today. She's still up and down with her weight.

Our beautiful angel is fairly stable, but she still has a tremendous amount of thick secretion in her throat.

When I arrived at the unit today Sofia was crying her little eyes out. I talked to her and stroked her tiny body to calm her down. I then asked the nurse to take Sofia out of the incubator for a snuggle with Mommy. Both Sofia and I loved it; we were in our own blissful little world.

Grandma and Granddad Vercesi visited today and Daddy came later on.

Daddy did Poppet's baby bed bath today and Little One just lay there proudly watching her daddy.

April 12—Fifty-eight days old (33rd week of gestation)

Easter Sunday.

Daddy and I received our very first Easter card from Sofia today. Inside the card was a tiny hand and footprint. Our daughter's!

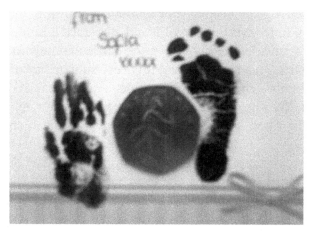

Sofia's actual hand and footprint against a fifty pence piece

Little One is now a massive 2.2 pounds.
Daddy did Sofia's baby bed bath today.

April 13—Fifty-nine days old

Little One had a big desat and brady again today and she needed "Tom Thumb."

Sofia is now at 2.3 pounds, which is good news.

I had a lovely snuggle with my baby and I changed two very dirty nappies and even got pooped on. Sofia also pooped all over her bed; she's like a little pooping machine. I love changing Sofia's tiny bottom. Daddy also ended up changing a very dirty bottom and had to use four nappies.

April 14—Sixty days old

Sofia is one seriously cute baby girl, if I do say so myself.

I did Sofia's baby bed bath and got peed and pooped on. We then had a really big snuggle and all was forgiven.

I took in a special baby dummy today, which had been sent from Aunty Charlotte who lives in a place called Rochester in America. Rochester happens to house one of the world's most prestigious hospitals. Aunty Charlotte was now a regular visitor at this hospital and every time I update her on Sofia's treatment and progress she goes and double checks that her little cupcake is having everything she needs. After introducing Sofia to the dummy, she had a little investigation of it and attempted a little suckle.

I have now learned how to move Sofia and how to put little vests on her. This is very scary. It is very strange having to dress your baby though the sides of an incubator. Because of Sofia's vulnerability she has to remain in her incubator at all times except for when we are allowed a sneaky cuddle if she is well enough.

Daddy changed a very dirty bottom and I tried Sofia with the dummy again later on; she tried her hardest to suck the end. The little madam will suck absolutely everything else, including her suction tube.

Sofia was weighed again today and her weight is now at 2.4 pounds.

Sofia and I had a little play in the incubator after Daddy left the unit, and I think Sofia could tell when I was getting ready to leave too because she started crying. I stroked her little body and rocked her to sleep through the side of the incubator before I could leave her.

Poppet is still having loads of suction and physio.

April 15—Sixty-one days old

Sofia is poorly today. She has had loads of desats and bradys and she needed lots of physio and suction again, as frequently as every half hour.

Poppet managed to have a sneaky little snuggle with me. Bliss.

Yet another very dirty bottom today, which to be honest is really good. A baby born as premature as Sofia can become seriously ill if she is unable to poo.

Sofia's feedings are now up to 9 milliliters an hour.

We had another little dummy practice again today.

Because of Sofia's bad day I was so worried about her that I went back to the hospital during the early hours of the morning. I just couldn't relax at home. Having to leave your baby each day doesn't get any better. It gets worse and harder to do.

April 16—Sixty-two days old

Sofia seems slightly better today.

Poppet's feeds are now up to 10 milliliters an hour. Can't believe it; it won't be long till she starts on pints!

I had a big cuddle today with Sofia, and after hours spent on the phone trying to locate a special face mask for his little girl Daddy had to drive to another hospital to fetch it. We are not impressed by this at all!

Sofia had a very dirty bottom again today and managed to poo all over me, her hands and feet, and the probe.

Poppet is definitely looking like a chunky monkey now. She looks like Les Dawson. She has really chunky chops and her little wrists and ankles are thicker too. On the end of those teeny feet are some juicy little fat toes.

I tried dummy practice again today but Little One was not interested. I think it is because she has such a tiny mouth. Sofia definitely likes sucking my milk from a cotton bud instead.

Becky Meechan

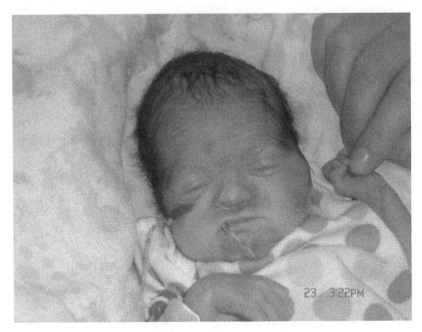

Our little Les Dawson

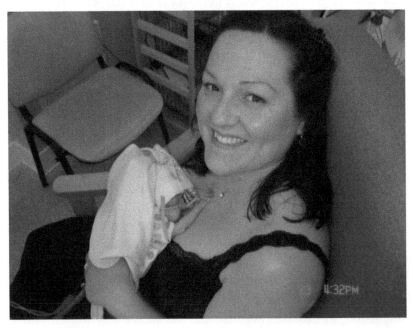

Mommy and Poppet

Nine Weeks Old

April 17—Sixty-three days old

Little One is 2.4 pounds today.

Sofia is still having desats and bradys. Will they ever stop?

Daddy and I both had snuggles today with Poppet, and she even had another little attempt at breastfeeding again.

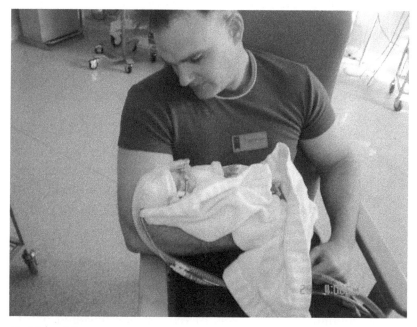

Daddy and Poppet

Sofia still has a very dirty bottom, which I am happy to see when I change her nappy.

Little smiles keep appearing and Daddy received a beautiful little smile from his girl today.

Sofia was a bit sick early on in the day, but she seemed to improve later on.

Today Daddy and I had a meeting with the consultants and ward manager. We are beginning to get very concerned about what we have witnessed in the unit and also some of the standards of nursing exhibited by various members of the staff. We have become very frightened for Sofia's wellbeing. Sofia has some truly fantastic nurses looking after her but there have been a couple that have worried us to the point of contemplating her transfer to another specialist unit.

The points we discussed at the meeting were as follows:

1. A senior nurse continually left Sofia unattended without any notification when she was moved to room 1 post-heart surgery and Sofia was very unwell. Sofia had a massive brady and desat and I couldn't stimulate her, and then I had to run into the corridor and shout for someone to come and help my baby because no one responded to the emergency alarms. I didn't write the date down of this incident but I told the doctors to check Sofia's notes to confirm the day in question when that particular nurse was looking after her.

   Prior to this incident I had continually voiced my concerns regarding Poppet's deterioration in health and these fears were dismissed. I was made to feel that I couldn't possibly know my own daughter.

2. A nurse had told me that Sofia had chronic lung disease. Chronic lung disease in premature babies such as Sofia occurs because their lungs are so underdeveloped that they are not able to function properly. On top of this, continually high levels of oxygen administered due to being on a life support ventilator for long periods of time hinder the development of their lungs too. I became very distressed, as the nurse was quite flippant with her explanation, and when Daddy and I questioned the doctors they told us that it was too early to confirm this yet and we shouldn't have been told in this way.

3. When Sofia was back on life support recovering from the massive incident on March 26, one of the nurses was continually away from the baby and also repeatedly coughed into gloved hands prior to handling the baby. This horrified me because I am a scientist and know only too well about transfer and persistence and cross-

contamination. This raised concerns as to whether Sofia's numerous infections have been caused by poor nursing practices. Sofia had three brady and desat episodes when this nurse was out of the room. This caused me to break down through sheer frustration and fear.

4. An incident occurred in the high dependency room on April 4 whereby the nurse kept wandering out of the room to chat to other nurses around the nursing station in the Bliss room. Sofia had a major desat and brady and turned gray and we couldn't stimulate her again. Yet again no one responded to the alarms and Daddy had to shout for help.

5. Staff from the delivery suite bringing a new mom into the high dependency room ignored the "wash your hands" signs. This is a simple and very basic hygiene requirement in an intensive care unit that houses extremely vulnerable babies. This is also a very bad sign of poor nursing practice exhibited throughout other areas of the hospital because if practiced correctly it would be done without thinking.

6. The inside of the baby's incubator was filthy for days, with dried milk residue on the internal walls. I asked a nurse to arrange for a replacement incubator because I was very concerned that the incubator was a breeding ground for bacteria, especially considering that its temperature was maintained at the ideal environment for bacterial growth and Sofia had already battled several bacterial infections.

7. A new care assistant came on to the unit (high dependency room) and continued to make unacceptable comments with regards to babies dying. I then had to tell her that my own baby is fighting for her life and she has made me very uncomfortable with her comments. The care assistant continually complained about the lack of induction standards and nursing practices exhibited by the hospital. I had to then explain to her how the monitors and alarms work. Again, this caused me to

become very distressed for my baby's safety and the quality of care she receives in our absence.

8. Information with regards to the baby's condition was not recorded on April 15. Sofia had a very bad day and suffered from a large amount of desats and bradys, which required increased suction and physio as frequently as every half hour. Yet this vital information was not documented. When I called the unit later in the evening to check on Sofia's condition I was informed that she would continue with her three hourly suctions. This prompted me to return immediately to the hospital because it was evident that the information was not passed on from the day shift, therefore other staff reading Sofia's chart would be mislead by the lack of information and may have thought that Sofia was faring better than she actually was.

9. Having no stock! This horrified us. How can an intensive care unit have no stock? On April 16 the unit had run out of small face masks and they didn't seem bothered. Daddy called hospitals all over the area in an attempt to try and track down the special face masks, and when he found a hospital that had them in stock we were told by the nurse in charge that they couldn't justify sending a taxi to the hospital to collect them. Daddy drove to the hospital in question and collected the two masks himself.

    Dummies together with specialist tiny nappies were another issue as well. Sofia desperately needed a dummy because she was "catching flies." We were told that Sofia was losing valuable oxygen because she was unable to keep her mouth closed. We were advised that the ward manager would find out the details of a supplier for us to contact. We heard nothing more. Luckily for us, Aunty Charlotte in America spoke to specialists in one of the hospitals near her and they generously donated some dummies for Sofia and her buddies.

10. Sofia's blood transfusions. I had to keep informing nurses of the air bubbles in the lines. I was told that there were filters in place and that the bubbles were too small to affect Sofia. However, one of the bubbles had already passed through the first filter, and because of this how could they guarantee the bubble would be blocked by the second filter? By then it would be too late. The incident in question occurred when I witnessed two bubbles measuring approximately 3 millimeters in length rushing toward Sofia's arm and one bubble approximately 16 to 18 millimeters in length was already heading straight toward Little One's arm on the inside of the incubator after bypassing the first filter. I had to urge the nurse to quickly intervene and stop the bubble. I want to know if nurses are aware of the mortality rate due to air embolism. I was so worried that I even contemplated contacting my works pathologist to ascertain the size of an air bubble needed to cause infant death. From this point on I specified that either I and/or Daddy always be present when any more blood transfusions were to be given. We just didn't feel that Poppet was safe anymore.

These incidents are not what you envision experiencing when you have a child fighting for her life, but we were becoming so frightened for Sofia's safety and care and we only felt relaxed when we knew she was in the care of certain nurses. This shouldn't have been the case at all. We should have felt confident in the care our baby was being given at all times, but instead we were falling apart because not everybody demonstrated a passion for their profession and the babies in their care.

April 18—Sixty-foud days old

Little one is 2.3 pounds today. Not good!

Sofia is a bit more stable today, but no snuggles. Although I did manage to do Little One's baby bed bath.

We are still having problems with Sofia's continuous feedings because the stupid machine keeps breaking, which in turn means Sofia is missing feedings. I am not very happy about this at all because she is not having her proper calorific intake. No wonder her weight keeps dropping! The doctors have put Sofia back onto syringe feeds at 8 milliliteres an hour.

Poppet lifted her head off the bed today when her blood was taken. She seems to be in a lot of pain, our poor angel. I would do anything to take her pain.

The doctors have put Sofia back onto sodium chloride and potassium to try and help her little body cope.

April 19—Sixty-five days old (34th week of gestation)

Sofia is 2.5 pounds today, little fatty bum.

Sofia seemed quite happy today, although she did have a number of desats and bradys. Fortunately most of them she self-corrected herself (meaning she was able to regulate herself again instead of needing help from the nurses and doctors).

Poppet was quite awake today and she liked having a little look around her den.

I was a bit worried at first because Little One hasn't passed any big poos since yesterday. I spoke to the nurse about it and told her I was worried there may be something wrong if Sofia's poo isn't any bigger because Sofia normally has dino-sized poos.

When I did Sofia's nappy change before leaving the unit, Sofia had one of the biggest poos I have ever seen! I was really shocked, but it does explain why she seemed to be getting a bit distressed, as Poppet hates a dirty nappy.

At the moment Sofia has gone to four hourly suctions and six hourly cares. The little rascal peed all over her vest.

Poppet stroked my arm tonight when having her nappy changed and then the sneaky little monkey wouldn't let me go home. Sofia likes me to stroke her to sleep and if I lift my hand off her she will wake up again and get distressed. This cripples me. I hate leaving Sofia when she is awake. I left later after I was certain Poppet was fast asleep.

April 20—Sixty-six days old

Little one is 2.57 pounds today.

Today Sofia had fleeting desats and bradys with a couple of biggies thrown in!

I fed and changed Sofia today and then got pooped on. She rested her hand on me again, and it seems that she is now trying to reach out and touch us. It is just the most beautiful feeling in the world to have those tiny little fingers flutter over your skin like a little butterfly.

Poppet and I had a lovely long cuddle, and Mommy has discovered that Little One absolutely loves her big toes being stroked.

Sofia really doesn't like being on her tummy and it really shows in her behaviour; a certain little lady increases her desats and bradys.

April 21—Sixty-seven days old

Today Sofia's best friend (another twenty-four-weeker) went off to another hospital for major abdominal surgery, as she is critically ill. Daddy, Sofia, and I brought her a little dress and a teddy to snuggle up to.

Little One is 2.6 pounds today.

Sofia is still having desats and bradys and she is now on suction every five to six hours. Plus she's still on lots of drugs.

Daddy and I had big snuggles today with our little bundle.

Poppet had her eyes tested again today; we have now been told that there is still the possibility of eye surgery for Sofia but we will know for certain in about two to three weeks.

Sofia had her first two vaccinations today. Daddy and I didn't realise that vaccinations are given the same as full-term babies.

April 22—Sixty-eight days old

Sofia is still 2.6 pounds.

Sofia is now having twelve hourly suppositories because she needs a little help when having a poo.

When I arrived at the hospital today Sofia was crying and so distressed. I had to cuddle her through the side of the incubator to calm her down.

Sofia's CPAP pressure has been reduced to try and decrease her CPAP tummy, which is extremely distended. It is called CPAP tummy because their tiny little tummies fill with gas and swell up like little puffer fish.

Poppet and I had a massive cuddle today, which was absolutely wonderful! There were lots of little tears today from my little angel, which breaks my heart. Sofia became distressed when her nappy was filled and also when the prongs up her nose hurt her. Sofia likes me to stroke her body and hold her tiny hands when she is upset and also when she is getting tired and dropping off to sleep. Sofia refuses to let me go until she is fast asleep. To be honest when those big eyes are watching me, it cripples me to walk away from her too. A mommy should never have to leave her baby at a time like this.

You can now hear Sofia's little cries when the incubator doors are shut. Her little voice is getting louder and stronger. Poppet also likes to make little noises when she is snuggling with me or Daddy. She sounds like a little baby croc, especially when she has hiccups.

April 23—Sixty-nine days old

Another one of Sofia's little friends left the unit today, but this time to go back to a hospital closer to home. We will miss him and his beautiful family. You naturally form close bonds with other parents when your children are critically ill.

Little One is now 2.7 pounds

It was a very big day for Sofia and me because we are now beginning our proper breastfeeding routine. It was our first real practice session and Sofia did really well. Daddy fed Sofia at the same time so that she could associate my breast milk with being fed and the sensation of having a full little tummy.

Sofia is still on twelve hourly suppositories to help her poo and she is now up to 9 milliliter feedings per hour.

Ten Weeks Old

April 24—Seventy days old

Sofia is now 2.66 pounds off CPAP and she has now been taken off biphasic CPAP and put on to normal CPAP.

Little One had a pampering session today and she had a little hairwash and massage from the nurse. Sofia's incubator is turning into a little beauty salon.

Daddy and I now have to feed Little One while she sucks her dummy. Again this is to try and get her used to feeding normally.

Sofia was quite awake and alert today.

April 25—Seventy-one days old

Sofia is now 2.75 pounds and she had a nice stable day today.

Tests have shown that Poppet's Co^2 (carbon dioxide) level is slightly raised, indicating that she might not be coping too well on NCPAP. However, her Co^2 level normalised overnight, which is a good sign because it means she may be showing signs of coping better.

Sofia is definitely taking to breastfeeding, but today she was sick at one of her feedings, which is probably due to too many medicines in her milk. This caused a desat and brady, which really frightened me. The nurse calmed me down and Sofia sorted herself out without needing help. Our clever little girl.

Poppet seems to be awake more now during the day too.

April 26—Seventy-two days old (35th week of gestation)

Sofia now weighs 2.73 pounds off CPAP. Her weight has dropped slightly.

Poppet's blood gas has been okay today.

Daddy and I played with our beautiful little baby in her incubator today. She was playing baby arm wrestling with Daddy, and I think she won.

Sofia had another attempt at breastfeeding; she definitely seems to like it. She then had a great big snooze in my arms and it was heavenly.

April 27—Seventy-three days old

Poppet is 2.71 pounds off CPAP today, again another dip in her weight.

Little One really does like to wake up during the day now, which is lovely. She just doesn't want to miss anything.

I had some dirty nappies to change today. Sofia seemed to be struggling with trapped wind. Her little face kept going red and becoming scrunched up, and those little legs looked like they were doing some sort of can-can dance.

We had another attempt at breastfeeding, but I think my milk is drying up now, which has really upset me because I have tried so desperately hard to keep it flowing.

Little One's smiles really melt my heart; they are so incredibly beautiful.

April 28—Seventy-four days old

Poppet is back to 2.73 pounds today off CPAP, which is great news.

Sofia had a couple of desats and bradys overnight.

Today was eye screening day again and Sofia is still at stage 2 of 3 (I understand that this condition is categorised as stages. Stage 1 being mild/none, stage 2 is signs of 3, and stage 3 needs laser eye surgery). Once they reach stage 3 the eye surgery has to be performed immediately in order to prevent blindness. Sofia's eyes are slightly worse than last week, but not serious enough yet to operate. Yet again it looks like Little One is going to have another operation. It is going to be a waiting game.

Poppet is now up to 10-milliliter (two teaspoons) hourly feeds to try and increase her weight.

Sofia is very alert and she is constantly watching Daddy and me when she is awake. We have discovered that a certain little lady likes to be tickled under her chin.

We had another breastfeeding attempt today, but I am not producing much milk anymore so Little One may end up being bottle-fed formula milk once my frozen supply has gone. However, according to Daddy this will be when Sofia is about twenty years old.

April 29—Seventy-five days old

Today was a very sad day. Our little family has been devastated by the news that Sofia's best little friend passed away during the night. May the beautiful little cherub rest in peace and may the angels carry her and protect her. God bless her. I don't think I'll ever understand how life can be so cruel. Our hearts go out to two very special families. Even though the little one lived such a short time on this earth she was a beautiful little girl who was surrounded with love from a family who we admire and respect so much. Words cannot describe our sadness and pain. We have shed many tears today.

Little Sofia has gained a little more weight today and she is now at 2.75 pounds.

Sofia seems to be tolerating CPAP really well, although she is still having desats and bradys.

Tomorrow Sofia will have her blood tested to check if her Hb level is okay and if there are any indications of Poppet's bone marrow (this is what produces blood cells) finally working.

Daddy and I held tightly on to our little girl today and thanked God that we could still hold her in our arms.

April 30—Seventy-six days old

Another bad day for our little family. I was called at 7:30 in the morning by one of the nurses who informed me that Little One has been very poorly. Sofia had a badly distended tummy and it is suspected that she may have necrotising enterocolitis (NEC). This is a medical condition primarily seen in babies born as premature as Sofia and it can be a life-threatening illness in which sections of the bowel undergo tissue death (necrosis). It is the illness that just killed Little One's best friend. How many more blows can our baby take?! Sofia has been put on nil by mouth for forty-eight hours. Sofia had more blood taken and she was put onto an antibiotic called Vancomycin (a drug of choice used in this situation) in case it is NEC. X-rays later showed that Little One's tummy is full of gas, which they think is mainly due to the CPAP. Sofia's CRP and blood gases are good. Thank God! This hopefully means no NEC.

Poppet became really upset during the afternoon and sobbed so hard. We aren't sure if it was due to the pain or because she is not feeding. Sofia was put on to her tummy and she settled into a lovely deep sleep.

Sofia's blood gas was so good later on in the day that her pressure was reduced and she was breathing air all on her own!!

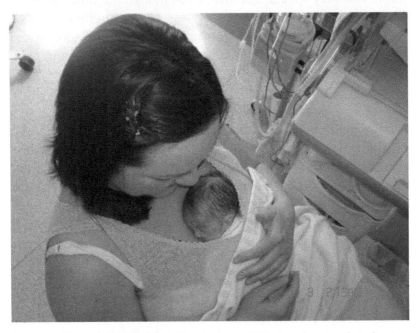

Sofia breathing air—the oxygen has been wound around my neck and tucked into my top facing Sofia.

Sofia is still having suppositories twice daily to try and aid her bowel movements and relieve the gas build-up. Poppet's tummy gradually became smaller toward the end of the day.

I stayed until Sofia was fully settled tonight. The last twenty-four hours have been very hard on our little angel.

Sofia's Hb is low, which is worrying Daddy and me. The doctors are giving Sofia time for her body to try and make its own red blood cells. Even though Sofia's Hb is low her oxygen saturation is really good (in the 90s, and she is on air), showing that she is coping well.

Poppet is now weighing in at 2.88 pounds. Yippee!

Eleven Weeks Old

May 1—Seventy-seven days old

Sofia has been more settled today, and her tummy is a lot smaller. She was still very upset again, but we think this is most likely due to the nil-by-mouth situation.

Poppet's poops are green, but this is probably due to Sofia not having any food in her body, which is causing her poops to be bile-stained (a chemical produced to help breakdown fats). The nurses used the terms "hungry poo" and "bile tummy."

The doctors are happy with Sofia today, which is fantastic news.

I had a very magical time today because I was able to express my milk at my baby's bedside for the very first time, which was lovely.

May 2—Seventy-eight days old

Little One is doing well. Her CRP is less than 1 and her blood cultures have come back negative so, knock on wood, no sign of a bacterial infection and no signs of NEC. Therefore Poppet's feedings have started again and she will be starting on 4.5 milliliters plus a drip to monitor her tolerance.

Poppet has very green poops but we have been told that this will change again in a couple of days once her feedings have gone through her system.

Sofia was a very happy little girl today with minimal support from CPAP. A very good girl.

May 3—Seventy-nine days old (36th week of gestation)

Big, big day. Sofia has been doing so well that she has been taken off CPAP. They have started her with one hour off first, then she will have two hours off, then four hours off to be followed by another four hours off, then another eight, then it will go to indefinitely. Scary! We have been assured that Sofia's blood gas will be constantly monitored.

Poppet is so beautiful and she seemed so happy to be free of all her tubes and hat. It was amazing seeing Sofia like this and hold her too. I can't wait to hold my baby for the first time without being surrounded by medical equipment and hospital staff.

Sofia's feedings have been put up to 8 milliliters an hour, and if she is tolerating them then it will go back up to 10 milliliters an hour.

Sofia's weight is 2.9 pounds. She now has really chubby hands, fingers, feet, and toes.

We are so proud of our beautiful angel and Daddy couldn't stop taking pictures.

May 4—Eighty days old

Little One is now approximately 3 pounds. She is massive!

Little Miss is still off all the machines and she is looking amazing. Sofia still needs suppositories, though.

I had a big snuggle with her, and both Daddy and I each did a baby bed bath today and both had very dirty nappies to change.

Sofia is still very pale, however she is showing slight signs that she is trying to make her own red blood cells. Another blood test tomorrow will confirm whether or not she is coping.

The doctors are thinking of moving Sofia back to our originating hospital if she carries on being a big brave girl. It is standard practice to return to your originating hospital once the baby is considered to be out of danger and strong enough to live without life support.

May 5—Eighty-one days old

Sofia has been a little poorly again. She had to have another blood transfusion so it looks like her body is struggling to make its own blood.

The good news is that Sofia is still off CPAP but her heart rate keeps dropping, which means she may be struggling to cope again.

Sofia's feedings are at 8.5 milliliters an hour and she is looking a little chubbier.

Daddy and I each did a baby bed bath. At some point we will have to learn how to bathe our daughter outside of the incubator.

May 6—Eighty-two days old

Little One is now 3.17 pounds.

Sofia's potassium level is low again, which is why her heart rate keeps dropping (potassium is an essential mineral needed for the proper function of all cells, tissues, and organs in the human body). Sofia is also being a little madam and she keeps closing her tiny mouth tightly, which in turn makes her heart rate drop. Cheeky monkey! That's yet another grounding! At this rate she'll be eighty before she's allowed out!

Daddy and I each did a baby bed bath, and I even managed to change Sofia all on my own.

Unfortunately we had yet more bad news today. Sofia needs to have laser surgery on her eyes. The eye specialist visited again today and Sofia's eyes have deteriorated rapidly and she now has to have surgery within the next few days. This also means that we cannot move back to our originating hospital yet.

Our poor little baby girl. Sofia is so beautiful and she has suffered so much already. When will she get a break?

May 7—Eighty-three days old

Poppet is fairly stable, although she has had a few desats and bradys.

We saw the eye specialist again today and the surgery has been arranged for tomorrow. A room will be set up for the surgeon to carry out his work.

We had big snuggles today and Sofia had more practice at breastfeeding.

Twelve Weeks Old

May 8—Eighty-four days old

Big day! Sofia had a massive cuddle with me before they took her away to be put onto the ventilator for her eye surgery. It was incredibly difficult for Daddy and me as we watched our beautiful angel taken from us again to be put back on to life support and heavily sedated. We sat with Sofia until it was time to start the surgery in the early evening.

The operation took about an hour and a half. Sofia behaved brilliantly throughout the surgery and only needed three out of the four doses of anaesthetic. Sofia was being given a drug called ketamine, which acts as a form of anaesthetic.

Little One is still on life support because her body is so full of drugs that she is not able to do anything herself. She will be on continual pain relief and needs to be kept away from bright lights. Sofia is to have regular steroid drops in her eyes.

When Little One's eye surgery was over she was moved back into the high dependency room, but her temperature was incredibly low. She needed to have a special heated gel mat to try and warm up her tiny little body.

Sofia's oxygen levels (sats) and blood gases are really good, which means if they stay this way then she can come off life support sooner rather than later.

May 9—Eighty-five days old

Things are bad. Little One is very poorly. She has not managed to come off life support and she is too weak, sore, and tired. Her tiny body just cannot cope with such a horrendous procedure. I became very distressed again, and I am now beginning to hate all the machines that surround my baby!

Our poor baby can only have minimal handling because it causes her too much distress.

May 10—Eighty-six days old (37th week of gestation)

Sofia is still on life support, but she has shown a very slight improvement.

Poppet is still very poorly and hates being handled. I managed to do a very quick nappy change.

Sofia's feedings are gradually increasing over time.

I was so exhausted today that I fell asleep at the side of Poppet's incubator.

May 11—Eighty-seven days old

A very, very bad day again. I was called at 3:30 in the morning. Sofia had had a bad episode, and yet again she had to be bagged. Apparently at 1:30 in the morning Sofia's feed refluxed, which severely affected her heart and breathing. Milk was found in her mouth and lungs.

Daddy and I headed straight to the hospital. Sofia had been put back on to a drip after several failed attempts to put a cannula into her. She even had part of her head shaved so they could try and put the blood transfusion through a vein in her forehead. This attempt failed and she now has a really big bruise. Sofia looks like a micro-sized Harry Potter.

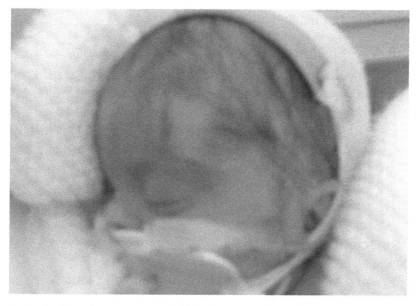

Sofia the day after we were called back into the hospital. The front of her head was shaved in an attempt to insert a cannula into a vein.

Sofia has been put back on to nil by mouth and she has had more blood taken as well as another X-ray. Yet again she underwent another blood transfusion.

Daddy and I became very distressed because the nurse kept leaving the spotlight shining right above Poppet's head directly into her eyes. Daddy had to move the light away and re-cover her incubator a few times to prevent Poppet's eyes from hurting further because of the bright light. Because of this Daddy and I later asked that this nurse not care for Sofia again. This was the second time she had done something which we didn't like. My nerves really cannot take much more now.

Sofia's tummy has been swelling again, but they think it is due to gas and nothing more sinister.

Sofia showed signs of gradually improving over the day, although she is still very drugged up due to the high dosage of ketamine she received.

Poppet and I had a lovely snuggle. I spent the day at her bedside and only left when the nurses made me go home to sleep.

Daddy came back to the hospital later on in the night and had a lovely snuggle with his little girl.

May 12—Eighty-eight days old

Poppet had had a good night, and when I arrived at the hospital today and she was back onto CPAP. What a massive relief!

Sofia was in a foul mood today because she had to have the nasal prong in again, which she absolutely detests! Fortunately after a while Little Miss was taken back off the CPAP and she has been coping without any breathing support.

I had another huge cuddle with my baby.

Sofia's feeds have been put back to 4.5 milliliters an hour.

Because Little One has improved so well she has been moved to room 2, which is a low-support room for babies that are less likely to have any scary episodes.

Sofia was crying a lot today; we think it's due to hunger because she has had very little feed over the last few days.

Sofia will have her eyes checked tomorrow to ensure the surgery was successful, and then if all is okay we can move back to our originating hospital. Too many worrying incidents have occurred now, and Daddy and I desperately want our baby out of this hospital.

Daddy went back to the hospital during the night to check on Poppet. We were worried that she now has less supervision and her little body has been through so much. Unbelievably, Daddy was verbally attacked while he was standing next to Sofia's incubator by the nurse we asked not to look after Sofia again.

May 13—Eighty-nine days old

When we arrived today at the unit Daddy and I asked for a meeting to be held with the doctors and matron in order to discuss the appalling behaviour demonstrated by that nurse last night. Enough is enough now! We are absolutely disgusted!

Sofia has been okay today; she is nice and stable, which is a good sign.

The eye specialist checked Poppet's eyes, but one of her pupils was not fully dilated so she will need a second check tomorrow.

Poppet is back on to full feedings. At last!

May 14—Ninety days old

BIG, BIG DAY!!

Sofia's eyes are okay so we can finally leave and go to our new home. At last!

Sofia was safely transported back to the hospital that we started at all those weeks ago. Yet again we had problems. Sofia's milk was left in the ambulance and the incorrect weight and information was sent along from the other hospital. The nurse receiving us had to call the transport team and request that the milk be sent back immediately, but it didn't arrive. Daddy and I got really distressed because Sofia had not been fed in over four hours. The transfer letter even stated that Sofia had had the full course of indomethacin before her heart surgery. I had pointed out this discrepancy to the nurses before Little One's journey but it was not amended. They even informed the new hospital that Sofia was on three hourly feedings, which she

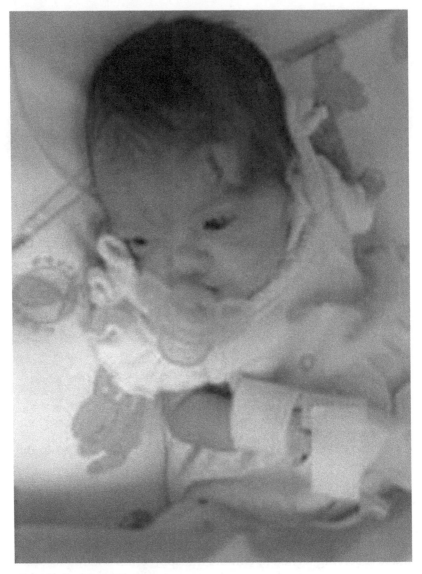

Sofia ready for the big move

had never been on. Sofia's weight was recorded from when she was on the ventilator and not off the ventilator, thus giving the impression that Sofia had had a huge drop in weight when her weight was checked at the new hospital. Thank God I kept a journal of most things. This horrified Daddy and me; we were frightened that Sofia's complications and battle for life had not been correctly documented on the transfer paperwork and future decisions could have been made by the new medical team based on the wrong information.

On arrival at our new hospital Sofia was put into isolation, or quarantine as I called it in the Special Care Baby Unit (SCBU). This was to make sure that she did not come armed with an army of little bugs. It is standard practice.

Because of everything that had happened, Daddy and I were worried about leaving Sofia at the new hospital. We had both lost so much trust and faith in the neonatal care system. However, we did have a pleasant surprise because at one point Sofia had a cheeky desat and triggered her alarm. Daddy and I were so shocked at the speed in which the nurse had run to our room that we couldn't help but smile. It was comforting to know that alarms are responded to immediately. I decided to stay the night at the hospital with Little One for peace of mind.

Thirteen Weeks Old

May 15—Ninety-one days old

My best friend Aunty Hayley (Bert) came to the hospital today to see her little "Titch" for the very first time. This was amazing for us both because only my mom, John, and Steve's parents had seen Sofia since her birth because of the previous visiting rules due to the risk of infection.

Poppet has really settled into her new home and the doctors have decided to try her without her suppositories, and thankfully she is pooing really well all on her own. Our big girl is showing us how clever she is now.

We had a little practice at breastfeeding again, which is brilliant, although I get very distressed in case Poppet doesn't like it because we have had only a few attempts in the past.

The hospital radio station played "Happy Birthday" today for Sofia to celebrate her arrival and then they played mine and Sofia's very special song, which is "Rule the World" by Take That.

May 16—Ninety-two days old

Pretty much the same as yesterday. Poppet has been behaving herself; she seems to be more settled here.

We had plenty of snuggles with our little girl and I tried another attempt at breastfeeding.

May 17—Ninety-three days old (38th week of gestation)

Fantastic news! I am going to move into the hospital and stay in a special room from now on with my girl. I am so excited. Even though we are still in a hospital and have a team of specialists around us, it felt wonderful to be allowed to live with my daughter at last and to start learning how to be a mommy and not having to ask permission to hold my baby anymore. We have our own little room and we sleep next to each other. Sofia's greenhouse is set up next to my bed so we can lie in bed and just watch each other. I am just so happy. I am grinning like a Cheshire cat.

Uncle Fez came to visit Little One today.

Poppet is on 20 milliliters of feed every two hours now, and she is tolerating it really well. Her baby bed baths are being carried out every six hours.

The next few days followed pretty much the same pattern and we learned to settle into a routine with Sofia and I living together and the three of us learning to live as a family, albeit still with medical assistance at hand. Sofia was moved to the next level of care and taken out of her incubator to live life as a "normal" baby. It was a very scary time for Daddy and I but also incredibly beautiful too because this was yet another massive hurdle that Little One had overcome. It also meant that we could just lean over her little plastic cot and cuddle her and not have to open doors to touch her. We had a few visitors who desperately wanted to meet our incredible little baby girl, including Aunty Lesley who is a scientist at the hospital.

I had stopped keeping my journal by this point, feeling that we were on the road home at last. However, after a few days

I decided to pick it up again and actually finish it when Sofia left the hospital for home. I resumed writing in the journal on May 26.

May 26—102 days old

Sofia's Hb is 9.8, which is fairly low. Not good at all.

We have not had much success today with breastfeeding. It is very disheartening.

Sofia is certainly a baby who likes to be cuddled and will quickly calm down as soon as she is held.

Little One is also a rascal when it comes to nappy changes. Today I changed a very dirty nappy and had just creamed Sofia's chubby bottom when she decided that she was going to do a poo on my fingers! Monkey!

May 27—103 days old

Sofia has had a few desats during the day and night. Nothing too serious.

Little One had to have her blood taken today in order to monitor her iron levels. They are still trying to hold off with yet another blood transfusion. We desperately need Sofia's body to start making its own blood.

Little One's weight is now a massive 4.1 pounds. She's not far off the 4.5-pound mark now. Yippeeeeeeee!!!

Sofia and I attempted breastfeeding again today, but I became very worried. I am concerned that Sofia couldn't get enough milk, which made her really hungry and distressed. I feel like I am failing her.

Sofia was tried with a 5-milliliter cup feeding today, which involves her sitting on the nurse's lap while a little cup is held to her mouth. Sofia then laps up the milk like a little kitten. It was such a beautiful site to witness but also very scary because I was so frightened that she would choke.

Poppet was started on folic acid today to try and encourage her bones and bone marrow. She needs all the iron she can get so she can have more wrestling competitions with Daddy.

May 28—104 days old

Sofia's iron levels are good today. Iron is needed for red blood production.

Little One had a desat and brady today but the doctors think it is due to her anaemia. They will continue to monitor her closely to be on the safe side.

We had a big breastfeeding session. Sadly we are not quite there, but hopefully we will make it between us.

Sofia had a little adventure today. She had a little go in a chair swing. Not quite sure what she made of it. I don't think she was overly impressed. Maybe next time we will have more of an idea if she likes it or not.

15 Weeks Old

May 29—105 days old

Sofia had her eyes examined again today. Knock on wood, things are still okay, but the eye specialist is still waiting to see what the blood vessels do.

We had some small attempts at breastfeeding today but Little One was so worn out from her eye examination that I didn't want to put any more strain on her little body.

Sofia is back on Gaviscon for her reflux.

May 30—106 days old

Little One now weighs a monstrous 4.5 pounds.

Our little rascal had a desat and a brady during the early hours.

Sofia and I finally had a stress-free breastfeeding attempt. Both Sofia and I lay down on the bed and snuggled next to each other while she suckled. It was magical. Neither of us became distressed. Then afterward we just lay next to each other while she continued to nuzzle me.

Later on in the day we had story time and I read a very bizarre Paddington Bear story to Sofia while she dropped off to sleep.

May 31—107 days old (40th week of gestation)

Today is Sofia's official due date! It is very strange for me knowing that my baby is 107 days old now, and she has never even been home or traveled in a car or any of the things you take for granted when a baby is born. When I reflect on what she has had to go through to survive, I still cannot believe it. We just cannot believe how quickly the time has flown.

Little One is still far off her expected weight had she been born on time. But who cares? She is still beautiful and amazing.

I bathed Sofia again today and got peed on big time. Little monkey. Sofia is still not sure what to make of bath time.

We had lots of breastfeeding attempts today too. Little One seems to be slowly getting the hang of it now together with me. We still have such a long way to go, though.

June 1—108 days old

Sofia went on an outing today. Only inside the hospital, though. I put a little hat on Sofia, which looked like a tea cosy, and then I pushed my tiny little chipmunk down to the X-ray unit in her portable little plastic cot. I found it quite strange when people stopped me to look at my baby and comment on how tiny she was thinking that she had just been born. Because to Daddy and me, Little One is huge now. When I tell people that Sofia is quite old now, the looks of amazement on their faces say it all. Our little miracle.

Poppet had to go for her brain scan to check if she has any long-term damage from all the bleeding on the brain she had and also all the oxygen starvation she had to the brain each time she stopped breathing. Thank God, all seems well. The specialist told me that Sofia's brain looked surprisingly normal given her horrific start to life. Yet again Sofia never ceases to amaze us.

I have had to make a very painful decision today with regards to Sofia's feedings. Even though I have tried desperately hard to keep my milk flowing since Sofia's birth, Little One is struggling to latch on to me long enough to feed effectively because her mouth is still so tiny. So after a long chat with the nurses I agreed it was best to start Poppet on bottle-feeding now too. I will continue to express my milk as long as I possibly can. Silly me, I became upset again when Sofia choked while I tried to do her first bottle-feed with a special pre-term teat. The teat caused the milk to gush and catch at the back of Sofia's throat. I really do feel so useless at times.

Unfortunately Little One's Hb has dropped to 8.5, which is not good all. However, her red blood cells have increased slightly, which indicates that she is now trying to make her own blood. The doctors will monitor Sofia overnight and decide the next step in the morning.

Sofia had a ten-minute attempt on my breast tonight, which made me really happy.

June 2—109 days old

Sofia now weighs 4.6 pounds, which is brilliant.

We tried both breast and bottle feedings this morning too.

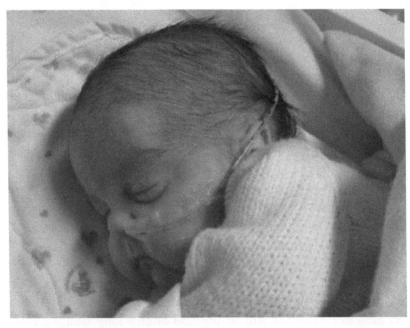

Sleeping Beauty

The doctors have decided to monitor Sofia over the next few days. They have decided to hold off with the blood transfusion for a bit longer, unless she starts to show signs of struggling. Little one is still slightly pale, but that is to be expected given her anaemic state.

I have noticed now that Sofia has started to show patterns of getting hungry and will stir about half an hour before her feeding is due. Again, another step closer to normalisation and away from a poor girl with controlled feeding patterns.

Sofia is now on a whopping 39 milliliters every three hours. It's a good job I made enough milk to keep a small country going.

June 3—110 days old

Little One had a good night's sleep and managed to drink two separate doses of 30 milliliters of milk from a bottle.

Poppet had a very distended tummy again today, but the consultants didn't think it was anything bad when they examined her. Most likely wind. However, they will continue to watch her closely.

Sofia's heart rate and oxygen saturation are both good, although she is still slightly pale.

June 4—111 days old

The eye specialist paid us a visit today. Little One's eye examination went really well so we don't have to have them checked again now for another three weeks.

I had some more attempts at bottle-feeding Sofia and they went fairly well, considering our history. Still not brilliant, but at least Little One didn't choke this time.

I had a fright tonight. Sofia was partially bottle-fed by me and then she had a tube-feed. But approximately fifty minutes later Poppet was sick and had a desat and brady, which resulted in her needing a bit of oxygen. The doctors examined her and found that she has lots of trapped wind. They have stopped the Gaviscon again and resumed the anti-acid and reflux treatments (Domperidone and Ranitidine). The doctors also felt that the bottle feeding is aggravating Sofia's wind situation. I became very cross and frustrated because the nurses all seem to have different opinions, which is not fair, especially after all Sofia has been through already. I keep getting frightened that I am getting it all wrong and that Sofia is just too weak.

So I will continue to try breastfeeding!

16 Weeks Old

June 5—112 days old

Little One is now 4.7 pounds.

Sofia has had a relatively good day today. However, there was a problem with the aspirate (pH testing) so they are going to have to re-tube her; it must be so unpleasant.

Sofia and I are now trying to combine breastfeeding and tube-feeding if she is awake enough.

June 6—113 days old

Today was a nice, steady day for Smelly Bum. That is, until I went home for the night. A certain little monkey decided to have a bit of a desat and brady about a half hour after we left the unit. But thankfully she then went on to have a good night. I do wonder if it was because we left and she didn't like it.

June 7—114 days old

Today was another nice and steady day for Sofia.

I bottle-fed, breastfed, and also tube-fed Sofia too. Poppet is still not too keen on breastfeeding; she sees it as a sleeping opportunity. Madam!

June 8—115 days old

One thing I can safely say about Sofia is that my baby can't half-poo! I now seem to be changing dirty nappies every couple of hours.

Sofia is now 4.8 pounds and on 45 milliliters of milk every three hours. I am happy to report that bottle-feeding is going really well; however, breastfeeding is not so well. Will keep trying, though!

Sofia's Hb is 8.4 so it has dropped slightly. We are awaiting the results of the red blood cell count tomorrow.

June 9—116 days old

Yet again more blood has been taken from Sofia. Apparently the red cell count failed yesterday due to the sample clotting. The new findings show that Sofia's red blood cell count has increased from about 2 percent to 5 percent, and her Hb is now at 8.7. Knock on wood, this means that Little One is now making her own blood.

I felt down again today because we are still struggling with breastfeeding. Sofia is very good at bottle-feeding but she still cannot handle the breast too well. We had a forty-minute attempt tonight at breastfeeding. It was reasonable; however, this was followed by a full top up from the bottle.

June 10—117 days old

I met the breastfeeding coordinator today and we had a very big chat about my confusion and frustration over all the different advice I am being given. I now have some nipple shields, which Poppet seems to like. They are silicone nipples that slip on over your own nipples in an attempt to help struggling babies latch on to you, which in turn enables them to feed better. They are as big as Frisbees. Not sure if Poppet has managed to get any milk through them yet, though.

Sofia's nasal gastric tube finally came out today after months of being fed this way. This is just the most wonderful news. We are now left with only one more clinical obstruction, and that is the monitor wire that is attached to Sofia, checking her heart and oxygen levels.

Our greedy little monkey had a right feast at one of her feedings and managed a whopping 70 milliliters of milk. We are now going to start waiting for her to let us know when she is ready for a feeding. That will either be a punch in Mommy's chops from a tiny fist or a cry. Again, yet another step closer to normalisation.

Little One has developed a very sore bottom. Some of her medication makes her poops very, very loose, and as a result of this they are irritating her skin.

June 11—118 days old

Sofia is now approximately 5 pounds. Whoopeeee!!!

Poppet is still bottle-feeding quite happily.

Daddy and I bathed Sofia today in a little bath bucket. We loved it, although Poppet is one slippery little rascal. She seems to really love having her hair washed.

We had a practice at breastfeeding with my Frisbee nipple shields today. Definitely not the easiest of things to get used to.

Sofia has been a lot more alert and she is a right little chatterbox, just like her mother.

Poppet's little bottom is still very sore.

17 Weeks Old

June 12—119 days old

Poppet still has a very poorly bottom. Now all you can see from her cot is this tiny, naked bottom sticking up in the air. We are trying to air dry her bottom in an attempt to dry the broken area of skin.

Little One has been very unsettled today, but that is possibly due to her bottom being so sore.

We are still trying both breast and bottle feedings and we are slowly making progress.

I am quite lonely tonight; I have no one to talk to. A certain little monkey is busy chasing bunnies in her sleep.

June 13—120 days old

It was bath day again today, and guess what? I got peed on!

Sofia and I are still trying really hard at the breastfeeding, and at 6 a.m. Little One fell asleep attached to Mommy. We stayed like that until 7 a.m.

Uncle Rob and Aunty Louise have given us their old travel system, so today was another very big day for the three of us. Little One went outside, exposed to the sun for the very first time!! We took Sofia for a little stroll around the hospital grounds. Aunty Carla took a picture of our very first walk together and after a number of failed attempts managed to only get the tip of Sofia's head in the picture. We laughed our socks off. Of course, once outside, Sofia, realising that this was a momentous event for the family, decided to sleep through the walk. The little bat! Poppet point-blank refused to open her eyes and held them tightly scrunched up. We did giggle. It was only when we came back inside the hospital that she woke up!

I need L plates on the push chair, as I am too busy smiling at my daughter and not watching where I'm walking. There may be a few dents in the walls around the hospital. Oops.

Sofia had her first hearing test today. Her right ear passed both tests but her left ear failed one of the two tests. We are not sure what this means at present, but they are going to repeat the test.

June 14—121 days old

Sofia now weighs 5.3 pounds. Little fatty bum!

Daddy and I took Sofia for another walk today around the grounds. This time Little One did a massive, stinky poo as a form of protest, and again our little bat refused to open her eyes outside.

Things are still not right with feeding patterns, but we are both still trying to find a happy medium.

Sofia definitely likes being swaddled. This is a method of wrapping babies up like little snug bugs. It gives them a sense of security. Our beautiful little caterpillar.

June 15—122 days old

It has been a scary day today. Little One has spent most of the day off her monitor. Daddy and I were a little concerned that it was for such a long period of time, but we have to learn to get used to living life without machines.

Madam is still trying to rip Mommy's breast off when she is feeding.

June 16—123 days old

Sofia still has a very sore bottom with very runny poo. It is looking incredibly painful and covered in open sores.

A little lady had a go on her activity mat today and she looked so tiny and cute.

We managed a twenty-minute breastfeeding attempt today without the Frisbee.

Sofia and I went for a little walk today around the hospital. I love being able to do something as normal as walking with my baby, and I just can't help but grin like a Cheshire cat.

A very special person arrived today. Aunty Charlotte and big cousin Jordy have come all the way from America. Aunty Charlotte had to visit on her own because Jordy was poorly. I cried because we hadn't seen each other for so long and because so much has happened. Aunty Charlotte finally had a massive snuggle with her little cupcake, who she thought she may never meet.

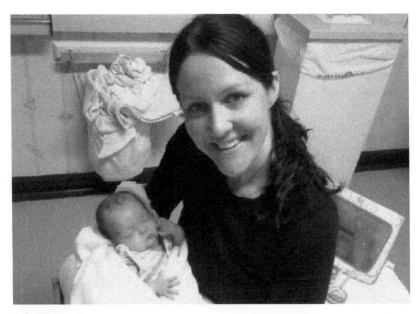

A proud Aunty Charlotte finally meeting her little cupcake

June 17—124 days old

Little One is now 5.4 pounds.

Poppet's little bottom is still very sore and her poo is so runny. I am getting very worried that she is suffering terribly. The sores are like ulcers.

Sofia and I went a little walk to the hospital shop today. We really do love this sense of normality and freedom. I still need to work on my pram-handling skills; we may have had a few more bumps.

June 18—125 days old

Sofia still has a very sore bottom. What is going to happen?

Not much change on the breastfeeding front today. Today was a fairly quiet day on the whole.

18 Weeks Old

June 19—126 days old

Sofia seems to have changed yet again. She is filling out more facially. She is beginning to look less fragile.

Poppet's little chubby bottom is still very sore but her poo is more formed now, which is a really good sign.

Sofia is averaging between 3 to 3½ hours between feedings, although she did try to eat Daddy today when they had a little snuggle.

It's funny the things you notice. Sofia likes to snuggle into Daddy's hairy chest; she's a bit like a gorilla in the mist on him and then when she is with me the little vampire loves to snuggle into my neck.

Over the last week Sofia seems to be trying to use her hands more and even appears to be trying to roll over. We keep expecting to see one of those little legs cocked over the side of her little box as she tries to make a run for it.

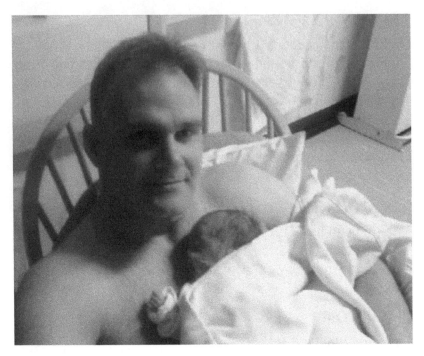

Daddy snuggling his little Poppet

June 20—127 days old

Sofia's bottom is still very sore. It looks like she has even more sores now. All you can see now is a tiny bottom stuck in the air most of the day as we try desperately to dry her wounds.

Poppet now weighs 5.7 pounds.

Granddad and Grandma Vercesi bought Sofia's cradle and Daddy has been kept busy building it today. It looks gorgeous and very much like one fit for a princess. White and frilly.

June 21—128 days old

Little One has spent most of the day with her bottom up in the air again, as it is still very, very poorly.

We are still practicing breastfeeding but it is very much a hit-and-miss situation. I really don't think that we will master this!

June 22—129 days old

No real change today; Sofia still has a poorly bottom and is still having to lie facing down with her tiny bottom stuck up in the air. It is just heartbreaking to see such horrific sores on such a tiny bottom.

I bathed Sofia today in a proper baby bath. It was the size of a submarine! I was convinced Poppet would be able to find Nemo in her little swimming pool-sized bath. One of the nurses helped me and we put some special oil in the water to help with Poppet's dry skin. Boy! Our girl can wiggle. Sofia absolutely loved it and she lay there like Cleopatra before trying the old walking on water trick. This is just so cute and funny.

Sofia's blood is okay today and no concerns have been raised. Again this is fantastic news.

June 23—130 days old

Sofia has put on .1 pounds today. I think she raided my sweets stash in the night!

That little bottom is still no better, and still not showing signs of healing.

I practiced my life support technique (CPR) on a special doll today. It was not the nicest experience in the world, but it is an essential requirement to have the knowledge when your child has been through so much already. Sofia watched me with those big wide eyes of hers.

Daddy has been testing Sofia's hearing today by whispering "monkey" repeatedly into her left ear.

June 24—131 days old

We had a visit from the wound care nurse today because Sofia's bottom is still very sore. Although, knock on wood, it is now showing signs of healing. Yet again the best thing we can do is keep that chubby bottom up in the air. Little One's poops are runny again so I had to do some poop-scooping for microscopy testing.

Little One had her third set of vaccinations today. She was not at all impressed!

Poppet rolled onto her side today, but only for a second. She's such a wild child. I have a feeling that this is a sign of things to come and my daughter will be a little fidgety bum.

June 25—132 days old

Oh my God, Sofia had her discharge examination today and it all went well. I can't believe just how close we are to home now.

We went for another adventure today and we caught the elevator down to the eye clinic in the hospital. Sofia's eye specialist is really pleased with her progress and, knock on wood, she is recovering really well from her surgery. Although, I could hear her little screams down the corridor as they performed the special tests inside her eyes. Sofia's next check is to be in six months. There is a possibility that she may be long- or short-sighted, but who cares? Any sight is better than none at all, and considering what our little angel has had to go through to survive it's nothing! We will face it together if and when it happens.

Poppet still has a slightly sore bottom but it is definitely showing signs of healing now at last. Those little poops are still loose, though.

Our little rolly polly keeps rolling from her back onto her right side now. It's like the great escape in that little plastic cot. Any minute now we expect to see a tiny rope chucked over the side and a little chubby bottom abseiling down with a backpack full of teddies.

It was bath time again today, and we put the special bath oil in the water again, which will hopefully help that little bottom heal. Poppet's Aunty Loretta and Uncle John came to see her today and she decided to be sick all over Aunty Loretta and me. It was not until later that I discovered that Sofia had been sick all over my bed too because Aunty Carla sat in it. Very funny indeed. My ribs hurt from all the laughter.

19 Weeks Old

June 26—133 days old

Little One's last full day in the hospital.

We have discovered that Sofia likes watching tennis and singing along to Michael Jackson!

Our little angel now weighs 5.9 pounds.

Little Monkey was showing off today, and while she was lying on her tummy she lifted her head up and turned to face the other direction.

Later on when Daddy spoke on the phone to a very grisly Sofia, she stopped crying and appeared to be listening to what Daddy was saying. Typical. She's clearly showing signs of being a daddy's girl already. Little monkey!

June 27—134 days old

HOME!!!!!

Finally the day arrives that we never thought we would see as a little family. Nearly five months after her birth, Sofia finally gets to go home with her mommy and daddy.

Our new journey begins . . .

Reflection

As I finish Sofia's story, I feel that it is important for me to address some of the issues we faced as parents in the hope that changes in the neonatal care system will be made for the better.

Unfortunately, our experience has caused me to lose a tremendous amount of trust and faith in our medical system. It became so bad for me that I wanted to fly Sofia to the States because I had lost all my confidence in the care she was being given here and was so frightened for her life. Yet I know it would have been an impossible task to achieve given her fragile state.

Such a high number of people gave up on Sofia even before she was born; even trained medical professionals talked to us in such a way so as not to encourage hope. My threatened miscarriage was handled with very little tact and compassion. Being told to return to the hospital the next day for a scan because the unit didn't work at night caused me immense anxiety and stress, both factors that have been known to contribute to the loss of a baby. Surely in this day and age and with advances in the medical field, it seems ludicrous to me that a hospital cannot accommodate such a procedure. A miscarriage, even in the early days of a pregnancy, is still a traumatic situation for a woman to face, and in the event of such a tragic circumstance the mental welfare of the mother should be taken into consideration.

When Sofia decided to make her early appearance and I was told by the consultant (when I began haemorrhaging) that my baby would just have to die inside me, it sickened me to the core. To me, it summed up just how ignorant people can be toward a family facing the potential loss of a child. It would be nice to say to these doubters, "Look at my baby now. You gave up on her and you were not prepared to give her a chance yet she runs, sings, laughs, cries, loves, and chats away ten to the dozen." Of course we know that Sofia is exceptional and her fight for survival is a true success story, but because of this attitude and the handling of my situation I was nearly convinced to give up on my baby daughter. Thank God I didn't, and most importantly I couldn't. How many mothers have given up because the situation has been handled so badly? Our experience has taught me that quite often there is very little compassion demonstrated by medical staff, and in particular by doctors. This should never be the case. It is a shame that some people let everyone else down. But sadly it only takes one of those people to completely shatter your trust and respect. The medical profession is one that requires compassion, support, understanding, and a nurturing nature. Yet to me it was very apparent that few people in this field appear to posses these qualities. It was also very apparent to me that some of the members of staff did the job out of passion and others saw it purely as an income. These differing approaches to caring for the sick make one hell of a difference in the standard and quality of care that is given. I feel the need to stress that we did have some amazing nurses and doctors looking after us; they were the ones we would go to the most, and they demonstrated all the qualities needed in an intensive care situation. We felt that the exceptional nurses in particular were undervalued and their dedication went unnoticed. So much can be learned from these nurses.

Initially, when Sofia began her fight for life, I ignored my gut instincts when I became aware of incidents that worried and concerned me, because what could I possibly know? The answer is, I knew my daughter. I knew her better than any of the neonatal team, yet I allowed individuals to dismiss my concerns and anxieties. One crucial rule I always abided by in a crown court was never to insult the members of the jury. I am no better than they are and I never presumed to be either. This is a lesson I feel many people in the medical profession could benefit from. A mother who sits for hour after hour at her baby's bedside knows her child no matter how premature her baby is. I feel that leaving parents out of the loop could potentially have an impact on the health of the baby. A parent may have made an observation that the nurses/medical team may not have picked up on. One such example of this was Sofia's deterioration post-heart surgery. Time and time again I voiced concerns about her deterioration, and each time it was dismissed. I was made to feel that my qualms were silly and that I shouldn't question the experts. I genuinely believe that the night Sofia had to be "bagged" for eight minutes could have been prevented if they had only listened to my fears. In a life-and-death situation there should never be a "them" and an "us." It is important to listen to the parents, take on board their concerns, work with them, and show them more support.

My advice to other mothers is don't be bullied into ignoring your instincts as a mother, because for generations women all over the world have raised children pretty well on their own. If I'd have ignored my gut instincts early on in my pregnancy, I would certainly not be writing this story now.

I included the list of complaints in my book not out of spite but in an attempt to heighten awareness of the damaging effects the actions of trained professionals can potentially have on parents. So many issues can be addressed and changed simply by communicating and listening to others. The staff involved in neonatal care need to recognise the impact that their care and attitude has on families.

I found it terribly demoralising having to ask permission to hold my own baby and then some days not being able to hold her at all. I had all the joys of a full-term birth cruelly ripped away from me, and I continually felt that I was a nuisance for asking questions or being seated at my daughter's bedside. I was not able to do the things that are taken for granted, such as smelling my baby, holding her against my bare flesh, being able to pick her up for cuddles, or soothing her when she was deeply distressed and in crippling pain. I know that this had a huge effect on my mental state of health, and it still does to this day.

It was soul-destroying each day to have to walk away from Sofia because I was unable to live with her. I had to tear myself away from my baby's greenhouse, and each time we were called back to hospital because Little One had taken a turn for the worse I couldn't help but blame myself. I would ask myself, *Would this have happened if I was here with her?* This might seem ridiculous, but to a mother and father who have to leave their precious bundle it is completely rational to think that way. I felt incredibly guilty each day when I left the unit. It was the most horrendous act for me as a mother leaving my critically ill baby and not knowing if she would be alive the next time I saw her. I began to become very anxious when I was away from Sofia and I couldn't wait to be back with her. I felt as though she was safe with me watching over her.

I found it absolutely appalling that an intensive care unit ran out of stock, which resulted in Steve having to chase down equipment and then being told that they couldn't justify sending a taxi to collect the required piece (a face mask). How can the neonatal system justify having a father call other hospitals because of no stock? We also had the predicament of it being down to the parents to track down specialist nappies and dummies. Thank God my sister lives in the States and sought help and advice. How much more insulting can you get to ask the parents of a critically ill baby to sort out and supply such basic hospital requirements? I ask myself, does the same principle apply to families of adults fighting for their lives in intensive care units?

On top of all this, I had the horrors of the milking cupboard to contend with. Surely a unit used to dealing with critically ill babies would know the importance of a mother being at her baby's bedside while trying to express her milk. But no, it appears not to be the case. I believe that if I had been able to express my milk at Sofia's bedside from the start instead of in a tiny cupboard at the end of a hall then I would have been able to have maintained my milk flow for a lot longer. I felt that I had let my daughter down because my only way as a mother to keep her alive was by providing her the best medicine that she could get. Again this daily worry was a burden that weighed me down mentally. Sofia was seventy-seven days old before I expressed milk at her bedside; all that precious time was lost, which could have helped my milk production. I feel that neonatal units should encourage expressing at the babies' bedsides to help the mommy both mentally and physically. It was soul-destroying having to sit in an old cupboard away from Sofia and sometimes having to wait for hours before it was my turn. Some days I'd be lucky if I got to express my milk twice while at the unit—no wonder I dried up.

I was horrified when Sofia was transported to the specialist children's hospital for her heart surgery and they rejected the bags of blood that were sent over with her. What if I hadn't been able to get there and provide blood in case an emergency occurred in the operating theatre? I couldn't believe it when I was informed that this was not the first time it had happened and that a number of incidents involving paperwork not being accepted had previously occurred. Yet they still had not attempted to resolve the matter and agree to a standardised blood transfusion form that each hospital is provided with. I simply could not believe that a hospital would waste such valuable blood. This didn't give me much reassurance in what was about to happen. How could I put my faith into a hospital that could not even accommodate the standardisation of blood submission paperwork? They really don't think of the impact this has on a parent. Not only that, but Sofia was severely anaemic and had to provide yet more blood, of which she had very little to give.

When Steve was verbally attacked at the side of Sofia's incubator by a nurse, we were astonished. The appalling behaviour demonstrated by a professional nurse again highlighted the poor standards of nursing practice exhibited in the unit. Parents have the right to protect their child, and if they feel unhappy with a member of staff then every attempt should be made to rectify the matter. There were days when we felt happier about leaving Sofia because we knew she was under the care of one of the "good" nurses. You should never be faced with that dilemma as a parent because all nurses should be demonstrating the skills that the good ones exude. We used to sit and wait to find out who was looking after Little One on the night shift before we felt it was safe to leave the unit and go home.

Initially we were too afraid to raise our concerns and challenge those matters that caused us distress, in case Sofia suffered as a result. We were not able to stay with her twenty-four hours a day, as the unit didn't have the facilities to accommodate long-term parents, so instead we bit our lips. It was only when we began to turn on each other and our nerves became severely frayed that we thought, *You know what? Sofia is our daughter, and to hell with them. We have concerns so they are damn well going to know about them.* But as it happens, once you start chatting to other parents in the same position you soon realise they have the same concerns and they, too, have bottled them up. I would like to say to the medical staff, put yourselves in an anxious parent's position and remember when you are all giggling around the nurses' station and appearing disinterested that you are being watched and your actions are affecting someone deeply.

People can be very clinical with you and forget that you are a parent facing the possible death of your precious child. The lack of care and attention given to parents and the frequent use of technical jargon when explaining complicated procedures or terms is not necessary. As Sofia progressed we found that we had to continually ask for explanations when the nurses and doctors spoke to us. I often felt embarrassed because I didn't understand or know what they meant and I felt unable to ask for an explanation, but fortunately for me Steve did ask questions. He was definitely my rock; part of me wanted to remain ignorant because I couldn't handle the constant feeling of humiliation. Neonatal units need to make more of an effort to provide parents with the understanding of the terms and procedures they use. It helps the parents feel more involved with their baby's care, and thus it takes away the feeling of inferiority when people all around you are throwing around terms left, right, and centre and you feel too embarrassed to ask what on earth they are talking about. A parent may have asked the same question several times over and they just simply haven't absorbed the answer. Please don't treat them as a nuisance, because they are people who are purely trying to cope with the horrors of their baby's daily battle for life.

When we moved hospitals and I found that milk that had been expressed in the early days had been ignored and consequently had to be discarded, I was devastated. After all my hard work and perseverance to battle to keep my milk flowing it was heartbreaking to see such precious feed thrown away because they were not able to facilitate the adequate storage and use of expressed milk.

Finally, when I began trying to breastfeed Sofia I became very distressed due to the confusion over all the different advice I was being given about the best way to do it. There clearly should not be several people all giving different opinions on the best way to breastfeed, because what this actually does is distress the mother so much that she feels like a failure.

The Journey Home

Where do I begin? Well, firstly there was the shock of finally taking home our baby girl, who at long last left hospital. Initially it was very scary. For over a third of a year I had been a mother to a critically ill baby who had never been home and had had a whole plethora of on-hand medical equipment and professionals keeping her alive. But now we were on our own. I was terrified of not having someone there to ask for advice and check if I was doing things right. I knew plenty of women who had babies, but apart from those I met in hospital I had never known anyone to have a baby born as premature as Sofia.

I remember being given a book to read by one of the nurses that I had formed a close bond with. She had found this particular book incredibly useful when she became a mother, and because I was anxious about coping in the outside world she gave me it to read. It was bloody awful. I felt as though I was putting Sofia through baby boot camp. Basically I understood it to mean that I should dictate to Sofia her sleeping and feeding patterns. It goes to show how just because one method works perfectly fine for one mother it isn't a given that this same method will work for you. After discussing my woes with my health visitor, it was decided that I go back to using good old fashioned, reliable maternal instincts. Which, I am happy to report, have worked wonderfully for both Sofia and me.

We were advised that we would now need to work on normalising our lives, and one of the consultants suggested that we cope without an apnoea mat, as it may be too disruptive. We chose to use one. The truth of the matter is for months we had learned to live with beeps and alarms and we had simply gotten so used to them that we forgot that they were there. Sofia settles each night and has always slept beautifully since she came home, so why remove that safety net?

We have faced so much over the last two and a half years. Sofia has attended numerous hospital appointments, which have included checks on her heart and eyes. She was also under the care of a dietician for her first year at home.

For Sofia's first two winters she underwent treatment for RSV (Respiratory Syncytial Virus). This presents itself as a cold-like illness in healthy children and adults. However, in the case of babies like Sofia who are born critically early and have spent a considerable amount of time on life support because their lungs simply cannot cope, this illness has the potential to make them seriously ill. Every twenty-eight days Sofia was given painful intramuscular injections into her thighs throughout both autumn and winter, the "wet" months of the year.

Sofia developed a very large umbilical hernia, which has thankfully reduced in size over time. Initially it caused her immense pain and distress and there was a strong possibility that it would need corrective surgically. Luckily it seems to be healing itself as the muscles in her abdomen grow stronger. Knock on wood.

Obviously, Sofia was born before my body could provide her with the kick-start immunity that mommies usually pass to their babies before their birth. She was severely compromised and at a higher risk than most of developing an illness, which she would struggle to fight. As a consequence of this, Sofia has had a couple of episodes that have resulted in her going back to hospital for a few days at a time. They were very frightening initially, but each time she managed to pick up and return home. Hence, for the first two years we exercised caution with Sofia and made an effort to keep her away from people with infections that are easily transferable. On the whole, she has done fantastically well.

We are about to face our first winter without any treatment, and to be honest I feel a little apprehensive, but I have to accept that this is part of letting go of the attachments to hospital and medication. A step closer to normalisation.

I'm not sure what I expected when I began keeping my journal, which is probably why some days are more detailed than others. In hindsight I wish I had included more information, but at the time having to write things down also meant having to go through it again and again, and I just wasn't mentally strong enough. When people say time is a great healer I now understand what they mean. For over two years I was unable to pick up the journal. I couldn't face it. I couldn't even watch any documentaries to do with premature babies on Tv and I still find it hard now; the beeps of a life support machine send a shiver down my spine. Even now when I look back at the journal I find it difficult and emotional. Only after my breakdown did I understand the shattering effects Sofia's birth had had on me. Throughout all the time we spent in hospital I battled endlessly as a mother to keep my daughter alive, and I was never able to relax because I knew that from one day to the next things could take a dramatic and potentially devastating turn. I was so driven by my sheer determination to bring home Sofia that I became almost robotic in my daily routine when away from her bedside. I hated being apart from her so much and I physically and mentally ached to be with her, touching her, talking to her, and holding her fragile little body against me tightly. It was only when Poppet was discharged from the hospital that I gradually began to relax into the role of a mother, but then unknowingly, slowly creeping upon me were the after-effects of the absolute devastation that had been inflicted on our tiny little family.

I have quite often heard over the years that having a normal, full-term birth can be a trying time for any couple, yet premature births bring with them such an immense amount of unexpected pressure that you literally feel your world turned upside down and inside out. Steve and I struggled immensely as a couple; we took it out on each other and turned on each other in our pain. Things may have been different if we had been given the support and help we needed at such an emotional time, but sadly we fought instead, taking our pain out on each other. Slowly over time we have begun to work things out, albeit with the occasional hiccup. We have been through so much together and we are blessed with such a beautiful daughter who completes us that we know we cannot walk away from one another, and neither do we want to. Alas, having a baby born life-threateningly early is a very intense time for a relationship, and sadly some couples don't make it. I understand why now.

When Sofia was born I made a choice, and that was not to turn my back on my daughter or give up on her. To my absolute horror, many did. This was so unexpected to me and also the last thing I ever thought would happen at a time when my daughter's life was hanging in the balance. I really felt my world fall apart all around me and I felt incredibly forlorn. If you would have asked me what I would have done had I been faced with a situation such as ours at the start of my pregnancy, I wouldn't have been able to answer because I simply didn't know. I took it for granted that I would be supported by those I loved dearly. I naturally assumed that they would be there holding me up no matter what and with them by my side I could face whatever life threw at me. Instead, I ended up having to face the realisation of just how cruel life can be and how quickly people abandon you when you are faced with adversity.

When I had my breakdown, I knew I could never be the Becky who once walked into a courtroom ready to take on whatever the judicial world threw at me; instead I began to suffer terribly with panic attacks and anxiety. I was petrified of being away from Sofia and not being there in case she took a bad turn. My nerves had taken one too many batterings and I could no longer put on that brave, confident face. Earlier this year I left my career on the grounds of ill health, due to my breakdown. I was sad to go but the near-death of Sofia many times over made me take a big, long look at myself and my life, and Sofia was it. I truly believe that sometimes things happen for a reason.

When I realised that I would be leaving work due to my ill health, I then found that I needed to make the most humiliating decision that I'd ever been faced with making and that was to declare myself bankrupt. The year 2010 was a year in which I hit rock bottom. I was so completely crestfallen. I had not only had a breakdown but I lost our home too. It became the year I made myself face everything head on. I sought medical help and counselling immediately, and to this day I still attend weekly sessions. Although I buckle very easily still, I have found that with each passing month I have become a stronger woman. I am fortunate enough to have the best medicine in the world, and that is my beautiful daughter. Sofia is my footsteps in the sand; she has carried me in more ways than I can say, and even though it's been incredibly hard the last couple of years each day I thank God for the gift he has given me. I also consider myself very fortunate to have discovered those who are truly beautiful in their altruism. They are the few people who share our lives to this day—the ones who never gave up on us and the ones who helped carry us through the highs and the lows.

I still have a lot of counselling to deal with, which I happily accept, because I know the only way forward for me is to confront my nightmares. If only there was more recognition and support for mothers of traumatic births then maybe no other mother would suffer the pain and emotional turmoil I faced. One day I hope society will speak out for its mothers; we may be doing what nature intended of us, but sometimes even the most natural act in the world goes terribly wrong.

Sofia (who is known affectionately as "Bub" from her bubble wrap days) is now two and a half years old and she has just been discharged from the children's outpatient department. Sofia's heart will be checked again to monitor the murmur and her eyes will continue to be monitored.

Sofia makes us giggle so much with her cheeky little ways and she is the most affectionate little girl in the world. Her smile lights up a room, and her constant chattering and tuneless singing along to her favourite songs warms your heart. Each morning my little daughter walks into Mommy's bedroom and climbs into bed for a big snuggle to start the day. Heaven. Sofia seems to be incredibly intuitive and becomes very protective over her mommy too. As I put together the final pieces of my book, I fill with warmth over the daughter I have been blessed with. Sofia is now about to start nursery school. Many moons ago this was a day we never thought we would see. Yet against the odds our

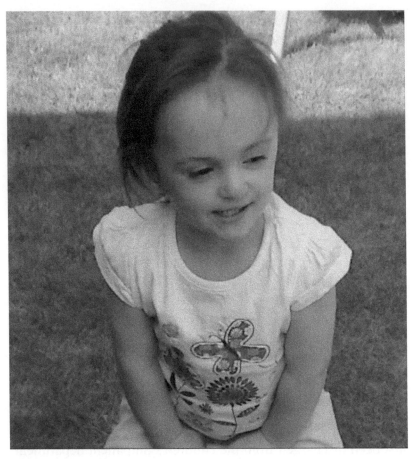

Sofia, aged two years

little angel will be beginning her next adventure in life, and I will stand proudly at her side watching her grow and develop and face life's adventures.

It is the most beautiful experience in the world to hear the words "Mommy" and "Daddy" or "Come on, guys." These are words we thought we would never hear from our daughter. We are truly blessed and never once forget how lucky we are. Our thoughts will always be with those who lost their tiny lives as they touched our hearts and our lives.

Final Words to Those Who Gave Up On Us

To the ones who turned their backs on us in our hours of need, to those of you who told others that our beautiful daughter would be better off dead because she would be so disabled and have no quality of life, and to those of you who broke my heart and tried to break my spirit: You may have gloated at my subsequent breakdown and bankruptcy, but even at my lowest ebb my daughter carried me through it. My beautiful daughter has survived against the odds and whether she had disabilities or not, never once stopped my love for her or made me turn my back on her. We have gone to hell and back many times over the last few years, but we never once gave up on each other. That is what happens when you have faith and a love that is so pure and simple. We will continue our adventure in life side by side and hand in hand, and my beautiful angel will never have to question my love for her or the sacrifices I will make to protect her from the pain and hurt you inflicted on me. I have nothing but pity for you all; you turned your backs on the most beautiful, most joyful, and most determined little fighter I have ever known. She is my life, my love, and my reason for living, my exceptional gift from heaven, my daughter, Sofia Angelina Vercesi.